Essential Calculations for Veterinary Nurses and Technicians

Essential Calculations for Veterinary Nurses and Technicians

Fourth Edition

Terry Lake DVM
CEO, BC Care Providers Association
British Columbia, Canada
Former Instructor, Animal Health Technology
Thompson Rivers University Kamloops
British Columbia, Canada

Nicola Green RVN
PMS Implementation Manager
VetPartners Ltd, York, UK
Former Veterinary Nursing Lecturer and Internal Verifier
Northumbria School of Veterinary Nursing
Newcastle College, Newcastle-upon-Tyne, UK

ELSEVIER

ISBN: 978-0-702-08401-0

Content Strategist: Melissa Rawe
Content Development Manager: Somodatta Roy Choudhury
Senior Content Development Specialist: Akanksha Marwah
Publishing Services Manager: Shereen Jameel
Senior Project Manager: Manikandan Chandrasekaran
Cover and Design Direction: Margaret Reid

Printed in India

Last digit is the print number: 9 8 7 6 5 4

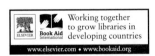

Contents

Preface

The veterinary profession, compared with human medicine, is relatively small and yet is quite diverse. We are responsible for treating many species of animals, and the response to medication can vary widely, making knowledge of dosage calculations extremely important. Veterinary technicians and nurses work with companion animals, food animals, research animals, wild animals and often no animals at all!

The mathematical tasks encountered are also very diverse, from calculating an amount of medication to give a cat to devising a quality-control chart for a piece of diagnostic equipment. These tasks are often the responsibility of the veterinary nurse and cannot be taken lightly as an error in one decimal place can mean life or death for the patient.

Although determining dosages can often come from consulting charts, understanding how these dosages are determined is very helpful in reinforcing other principles in physiology, pathology and case management. In some situations, you will need to create a dosage chart for your practice and hopefully this book will provide you with all the tools required.

This book relies heavily on dimensional analysis, a method of converting units from one form to another by using conversion factors as 'bridges'. You may recall this method in chemistry courses. It eliminates the necessity of memorizing formulae and takes advantage of simplifying equations so that calculators are often unnecessary. Not everyone takes to this technique, however, so other methods, such as ratio and proportion, are also described.

Although students in veterinary nursing courses have been taught basic arithmetical concepts prior to enrolling in the program, it is often the case that a review is needed to recall them. We have come to rely so heavily on calculators that skills such as long division and working with scientific notation are quickly lost. It is important to understand how these calculations are performed so that we can work in the absence of a calculator or at least recognize when we may have punched the wrong button.

The student resources on this book's accompanying Evolve website now include a wealth of additional practice questions to help students master key mathematical concepts. Instructors will find PowerPoint lectures and answers to students' practice questions, as well as a robust test bank with more than 250 questions.

You will find your veterinary nursing program exciting and challenging and I hope that even if Maths is not your favourite course, this book will build your confidence in calculating dosages for your patients.

Terry Lake
British Columbia, 2021

Chapter 1

Review of basic maths

Learning Objectives

- What is a fraction?
- Types of fraction

- How to convert and reduce fractions
- Finding the lowest common denominator
- How to add, subtract, multiply and divide fractions
- What are decimals and percentages?
- The importance of zeros
- How to add and subtract decimals
- How to multiply and divide decimals
- How to round off decimals
- Converting fractions to decimals
- Converting decimals to fractions
- How to add and subtract percentages
- How to multiply and divide percentages
- What is scientific notation?
- How to express numbers in scientific notation
- How to multiply and divide in scientific notation
- How to add and subtract in scientific notation

What is a fraction?

When something is divided into equal parts, each part represents a fraction of the whole. The number of equal parts in the whole represents the denominator (lower figure in the fraction) and the number of parts being considered represents the numerator (upper figure). If a pie is cut into 8 equal pieces (the number of pieces in the whole pie) and 3 are eaten (the number of pieces being considered), we can say $\frac{3}{8}$ of the pie has been eaten.

A fraction allows us to consider a number of parts in relation to the whole. This may be a number smaller than the whole, as in the example above, in which case this is a proper fraction. We can also consider a fraction that is greater than the whole – an improper fraction. If I had 2 pies, each divided into 8 equal pieces, and 13 pieces were eaten, $\frac{13}{8}$ of a pie have been consumed. An improper fraction can also be expressed as a mixed number – a whole number and a proper fraction. In our example, $1\frac{5}{8}$ of a pie has been eaten (one whole pie plus five eighths of a second pie).

Converting fractions

Converting mixed numbers to improper fractions makes it easier for us to work with fractions. This conversion involves two steps:

● Multiply the denominator by the whole number
● Add the numerator.

The denominator stays the same.

$1\dfrac{5}{8}$ becomes: $8 \times 1 = 8 \longrightarrow 8 + 5 = 13 \longrightarrow \dfrac{13}{8}$

 Let's do it again!

Convert the following mixed numbers to improper fractions.

1. $2\dfrac{3}{7}$ 2. $6\dfrac{3}{4}$ 3. $21\dfrac{8}{9}$ 4. $8\dfrac{2}{3}$ 5. $3\dfrac{5}{8}$

ANSWERS

1. $\dfrac{17}{7}$ 2. $\dfrac{27}{4}$ 3. $\dfrac{197}{9}$ 4. $\dfrac{26}{3}$ 5. $\dfrac{29}{8}$

Of course we can convert improper fractions into mixed numbers by doing the reverse:

● Divide the numerator by the denominator
● The amount 'left over' becomes the new numerator.

$\dfrac{23}{6}$ becomes: $23 \div 6 = 3$, with 5 left over $\rightarrow 3\dfrac{5}{6}$

 Let's do it again!

Convert the following improper fractions to mixed numbers.

1. $\dfrac{13}{7}$ 2. $\dfrac{25}{9}$ 3. $\dfrac{47}{6}$ 4. $\dfrac{17}{8}$ 5. $\dfrac{19}{10}$

ANSWERS

1. $1\dfrac{6}{7}$ 2. $2\dfrac{7}{9}$ 3. $7\dfrac{5}{6}$ 4. $2\dfrac{1}{8}$ 5. $1\dfrac{9}{10}$

Reducing fractions

Reducing a fraction means converting a fraction to produce the smallest numbers possible in the numerator and denominator and is also known as simplifying a fraction because why say $\frac{4}{8}$ of a pie when you can say $\frac{1}{2}$? Simplifying a fraction is accomplished by dividing the numerator and denominator by the largest common number possible.

$$\frac{10}{12} \text{ becomes: } \frac{10 \div 2}{12 \div 2} = \frac{5}{6}$$

This operation demonstrates an important concept: if you multiply or divide the numerator and the denominator by the same number, you do not change the value of the fraction, only its appearance. This is because you are simply multiplying or dividing the fraction by 1. In this example, we have divided both the numerator and denominator by 2, or if we consider the fraction, we have divided the fraction by $\frac{2}{2}$, which is of course 1.

Let's do it again!

Reduce the following fractions to their lowest terms.

1. $\frac{6}{8}$ 2. $\frac{4}{12}$ 3. $\frac{125}{500}$ 4. $\frac{64}{22}$ 5. $\frac{21}{56}$

ANSWERS

1. $\frac{3}{4}$ 2. $\frac{1}{3}$ 3. $\frac{1}{4}$ 4. $\frac{32}{11}$ 5. $\frac{3}{8}$

Finding the common denominator

There are times when we need to make different fractions look similar so that we can work with them. This is called finding the common denominator. This is most easily done by multiplying all the denominators in a set of fractions.

For $\frac{3}{8}$ and $\frac{5}{6}$, the common denominator is 48 (8 × 6 = 48)

Then multiply each numerator by the same number as its denominator: 8 goes into 48 6 times, so we multiply 3 by 6 to give us $18 \longrightarrow \frac{18}{48} \left(\frac{3}{8}\right)$.

6 goes into 48 8 times, so we multiply 5 by 8 to give us

$$40 \longrightarrow \frac{40}{48} \left(\frac{5}{6} \right).$$

The lowest common denominator (LCD) is the smallest number that is a multiple of all the denominators in a set of fractions. In our example above, 24 is the LCD, so $\frac{3}{8}$ can be expressed as $\frac{9}{24}$ and $\frac{5}{6}$ can be expressed as $\frac{20}{24}$.

Finding the LCD is not always easy, so we must have a method to help us. Consider the set of fractions: $\frac{1}{2}$, $\frac{2}{3}$, $\frac{5}{6}$ and $\frac{4}{9}$. The LCD is not obvious, so use this technique:

1. Place all the denominators in a line from lowest to highest: 2 3 6 9.
2. Divide the numbers by the smallest number that will go into at least two of them.
3. Bring down all the numbers that cannot be divided.
4. Continue until all denominators are reduced to one:

$$2\ 3\ 6\ 9$$

Divide by 2 $\longrightarrow$ 1 3 3 9

Divide by 3 $\longrightarrow$ 1 1 1 3

Divide by 3 $\longrightarrow$ 1 1 1 1

5. Now multiply the numbers you used to divide: $2 \times 3 \times 3 = 18$. The LCD is 18.

The set of fractions now becomes:

$$\frac{1}{2} = \frac{9}{18}, \ \frac{2}{3} = \frac{12}{18}, \ \frac{5}{6} = \frac{15}{18}, \ \frac{4}{9} = \frac{8}{18}$$

 Let's do it again!

Find the LCD for each set of fractions.

1. $\frac{3}{5}, \frac{4}{7}, \frac{5}{9}, \frac{3}{10}$ 2. $\frac{2}{3}, \frac{5}{6}, \frac{5}{12}, \frac{5}{9}$ 3. $\frac{4}{21}, \frac{3}{7}, \frac{4}{9}$ 4. $\frac{11}{12}, \frac{3}{4}, \frac{5}{6}$

ANSWERS

1. 630   2. 36   3. 63   4. 12

Converting dissimilar fractions into fractions with LCD makes comparing fractions much easier. This can help when deciding which medication strength is higher.

Using tablets of equal strength, is $\frac{4}{5}$ of a tablet more than $\frac{6}{7}$ of a tablet?

LCD = 35, so $\frac{4}{5}$ becomes $\frac{28}{35}$ and $\frac{6}{7}$ becomes $\frac{30}{35}$

Therefore, $\frac{6}{7}$ is greater than $\frac{4}{5}$.

 Remember: When comparing fractions with common denominators, the fraction with the largest numerator is the largest number.

Adding and subtracting fractions

We have seen that it is sometimes difficult to compare dissimilar fractions (think of it like trying to compare apples to oranges). Converting fractions to the LCD is a great way to allow us to compare apples with apples. When adding and subtracting fractions, we must convert them to the LCD because we cannot add dissimilar things, i.e. we cannot add apples to oranges (Fig. 1.1)!

To add fractions:

1. First find the LCD
2. Express each fraction using the LCD
3. Add the numerators
4. Convert to a mixed number if necessary.

$$\frac{2}{3} + \frac{3}{4} \longrightarrow LCD = 12$$

$$\frac{2}{3} = \frac{8}{12}, \frac{3}{4} = \frac{9}{12}$$

$$\frac{8}{12} + \frac{9}{12} = \frac{17}{12} = 1\frac{5}{12}$$

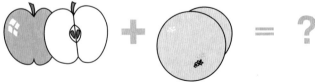

Fig. 1.1 Dissimilar things or units cannot be added together

To subtract fractions:
1. First find the LCD
2. Express each fraction using the LCD
3. Subtract the numerators
4. Convert to a mixed number if necessary.

$$1\frac{3}{4} - \frac{5}{6} \longrightarrow LCD = 12$$

$$1\frac{3}{4} = \frac{7}{4} = \frac{21}{12}, \frac{5}{6} = \frac{10}{12}$$

$$\frac{21}{12} - \frac{10}{12} = \frac{11}{12}$$

 ## Let's do it again!

1. $\frac{2}{3} + \frac{5}{6}$ 2. $\frac{5}{7} + \frac{3}{5}$ 3. $\frac{7}{12} + \frac{3}{4} + \frac{3}{8}$ 4. $\frac{21}{25} + \frac{3}{5} + \frac{7}{15}$ 5. $\frac{8}{9} + \frac{2}{3}$

6. $\frac{11}{12} - \frac{2}{3}$ 7. $\frac{7}{8} - \frac{5}{6}$ 8. $\frac{23}{6} - \frac{3}{4}$ 9. $\frac{9}{11} - \frac{2}{3}$ 10. $\frac{65}{5} - \frac{1}{10}$

ANSWERS

1. $1\frac{1}{2}$ 2. $1\frac{11}{35}$ 3. $1\frac{17}{24}$ 4. $1\frac{68}{75}$ 5. $1\frac{5}{9}$ 6. $\frac{1}{4}$ 7. $\frac{1}{24}$ 8. $3\frac{1}{12}$

9. $\frac{5}{33}$ 10. $12\frac{9}{10}$

Multiplying fractions

Unlike adding and subtracting, we do not need to find the LCD when multiplying or dividing fractions. The numerator of one fraction is multiplied by the numerator of the second fraction, and the denominator of the first is multiplied by the denominator of the second:

$$\frac{2}{3} \times \frac{4}{5} \longrightarrow \frac{2 \times 4}{3 \times 5} = \frac{8}{15}$$

If a fraction is multiplied by a whole number, think of the whole number as a fraction with 1 as the denominator:

$$\frac{2}{3} \times 4 \longrightarrow \frac{2 \times 4}{3 \times 1} = \frac{8}{3} \longrightarrow \frac{8}{3} = 2\frac{2}{3}$$

If multiplying mixed numbers, convert them to improper fractions before multiplying:

$$3\frac{4}{5} \times 12\frac{6}{7} \longrightarrow \frac{19}{5} \times \frac{90}{7} \longrightarrow \frac{19 \times 90}{5 \times 7} = \frac{1710}{35} = 48\frac{30}{35} = 48\frac{6}{7}$$

 Let's do it again!

Multiply the following fractions.

1. $\frac{3}{7} \times \frac{5}{6}$ 2. $\frac{13}{4} \times \frac{2}{3}$ 3. $1\frac{2}{5} \times 4\frac{5}{6}$ 4. $\frac{9}{11} \times 4\frac{3}{4}$ 5. $\frac{21}{6} \times 3\frac{2}{3}$

ANSWERS

1. $\frac{15}{42} = \frac{5}{14}$ 2. $2\frac{1}{6}$ 3. $6\frac{23}{30}$ 4. $3\frac{39}{44}$ 5. $12\frac{5}{6}$

Dividing fractions

As in multiplication, we can divide fractions without worrying about converting them to their LCD. To divide fractions, simply invert the divisor (the number doing the dividing) and multiply:

$$\frac{2}{3} \div \frac{4}{5} \longrightarrow \frac{2}{3} \times \frac{5}{4} = \frac{10}{12} = \frac{5}{6}$$

To convince yourself that it is okay to do this inversion, consider one half of a pie that was to be shared by two people – in other words, the $\frac{1}{2}$ of a pie was divided by 2. You intuitively know that each person would receive $\frac{1}{4}$ of the pie, but this is how it would look (remember that $\frac{2}{1}$ is the same as 2):

$$\frac{1}{2} \div \frac{2}{1} \longrightarrow \frac{1}{2} \times \frac{1}{2} \left(\text{i.e. we have inverted } \frac{2}{1} \right) = \frac{1}{4}$$

 Remember to convert mixed numbers to improper fractions before dividing.

 # Let's do it again!

Divide the following fractions.

1. $\frac{3}{7} \div \frac{5}{6}$ 2. $\frac{13}{4} \div \frac{2}{3}$ 3. $1\frac{2}{5} \div 4\frac{5}{6}$ 4. $\frac{9}{11} \div 4\frac{3}{4}$ 5. $\frac{22}{6} \div 3\frac{2}{3}$

ANSWERS

1. $\frac{18}{35}$ 2. $4\frac{7}{8}$ 3. $\frac{42}{145}$ 4. $\frac{36}{209}$ 5. 1

Complex fractions

A fraction in which either the numerator or denominator, or both, are themselves fractions is called a complex fraction. Since the line between the numerator and the denominator really means divided by, a complex fraction is simply one fraction divided by another. Remember, when dividing fractions, invert the second fraction and multiply.

$$\frac{\dfrac{2}{3}}{\dfrac{3}{4}} = \frac{2}{3} \div \frac{3}{4} \longrightarrow \frac{2}{3} \times \frac{4}{3} = \frac{8}{9}$$

Let's do it again!

Solve the following complex fractions.

1. $\dfrac{\frac{4}{5}}{\frac{1}{2}}$ 2. $\dfrac{\frac{13}{5}}{\frac{3}{4}}$ 3. $\dfrac{\frac{8}{9}}{\frac{3}{7}}$ 4. $\dfrac{\frac{2}{5}}{\frac{5}{2}}$ 5. $\dfrac{\frac{22}{7}}{\frac{3}{2}}$

ANSWERS

1. $1\frac{3}{5}$ 2. $3\frac{7}{15}$ 3. $2\frac{2}{27}$ 4. $\frac{4}{25}$ 5. $2\frac{2}{21}$

What is a decimal?

A decimal is simply a fraction in which the denominator is 10 or a power of 10 (*deci* is a Latin root word that means one tenth, $\frac{1}{10}$). Instead of writing a fraction, we can express the denominator by using a *decimal point*. In this way, $\frac{1}{10}$ becomes 0.1. If we wanted to express the fraction $\frac{4}{10}$ as a decimal, it would appear as 0.4. The denominator in a decimal fraction can be any power of 10: 10, 100, 1000, 10,000, etc. Each power of 10 has a place to the right of the decimal point for proper fractions, whereas each whole number with a power of 10 has a place to the left of the decimal point (Fig. 1.2).

Using this system, any number with a denominator that has a power of 10 can be expressed as a decimal: $\frac{12}{100}$ becomes 0.12, $\frac{125}{1000}$ becomes 0.125, $\frac{32,456}{10,000}$ becomes 3.2456.

Zero in on zeros!

It is very important to include the zero to the left of the decimal point in numbers less than 1. Imagine reading a medication order for a dog that states: 'Give .1 mg intravenously every 8 hours'. The decimal point may be lost, especially with the notoriously poor penmanship of veterinarians. It may be read as: 'Give 1 mg intravenously every 8 hours', resulting in a 10 times overdosage! The correct way to write the order is: 'Give 0.1 mg intravenously every 8 hours'.

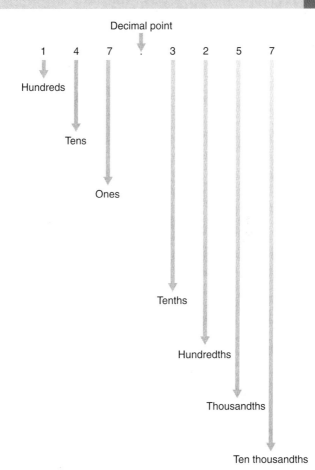

Fig. 1.2 Powers of 10 on either side of the decimal point

Same safety idea as the leading zero: 3.0 mg can easily be read as 30 mg. Always a leading zero, never a trailing zero! When zeros to the *right* of the decimal point do not appear in front of other numbers, they can be eliminated, e.g. 3.4500 can be written 3.45. The number 3.4507 must, of course, retain its zero.

Let's do it again!

Express the following fractions as decimals.

1. $\frac{33}{100}$ 2. $\frac{345}{1000}$ 3. $\frac{25}{10,000}$ 4. $\frac{35}{10}$ 5. $\frac{8}{100}$

ANSWERS

1. 0.33   2. 0.345   3. 0.0025   4. 3.5   5. 0.08

Working with decimals

Adding and subtracting decimals

The only trick here is to line up the decimals correctly to ensure proper placement. It is a good idea to use zeros (appropriately, of course) to help you line up the numbers:

$$
\begin{array}{r}
1.234 \\
+\ 0.310 \\
\hline
1.544
\end{array}
\qquad
\begin{array}{r}
0.035 \\
+\ 5.600 \\
\hline
5.635
\end{array}
\qquad
\begin{array}{r}
12.0020 \\
-\ 0.1235 \\
\hline
11.8785
\end{array}
$$

Multiplying decimals

No need to line up decimal points with multiplication of decimals. The trick here is to ensure you have the correct number of decimal places in the product. This should equal the sum of the decimal places in the two numbers being multiplied.

$$
\begin{array}{r}
5.5 \\
\times\quad 0.125 \\
\hline
0.6875
\end{array}
$$

→ 1 decimal place from right
→ 3 decimal places from right
→ 4 decimal places (1 + 3)

$$
\begin{array}{r}
10.75 \\
\times\quad 5.0005 \\
\hline
53.755375
\end{array}
$$

Dividing decimals

The number that is being divided is called the *dividend*, whereas the number doing the dividing is called the *divisor*. The number that results is called the *quotient*.

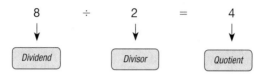

$$8 \qquad \div \qquad 2 \qquad = \qquad 4$$

Dividend   Divisor   Quotient

When the divisor is a whole number, simply place the quotient's decimal point in the same place it appeared in the dividend:

$$\begin{array}{r} 5.3 \\ 2\overline{)10.6} \end{array} \qquad \begin{array}{r} 0.8052 \\ 125\overline{)100.6500} \end{array}$$

If the divisor and the dividend are both decimals, we must convert the divisor to a whole number first. This is done by moving the decimal point of the divisor as far to the right as needed to get rid of it and then moving the dividend's decimal point the same number of places.

$$1.5\overline{)10.05} \longrightarrow 15\overline{)100.5} \longrightarrow \begin{array}{r} 6.7 \\ 15\overline{)100.5} \end{array}$$

$$0.005\overline{)100.1} \longrightarrow 5\overline{)100,100} \longrightarrow \begin{array}{r} 20,020 \\ 5\overline{)100,100} \end{array}$$

In the last example, we had to add 2 zeros at the end of the dividend in order to move the decimal point over 3 places – the number of places it was moved to make the divisor a whole number.

Let's do it again!

Multiply or divide the following decimals.

1. 4.5×6.75 2. 0.1×45.5 3. 12.075×0.01

4. 5.01×100.25 5. 3.5×1.005 6. $5.05 \div 2$

7. $10.75 \div 0.05$ 8. $100 \div 0.002$ 9. $\frac{10.8}{2.4}$ 10. $\frac{0.75}{5}$

ANSWERS

1. 30.375   2. 4.55   3. 0.12075   4. 502.2525   5. 3.5175

6. 2.525   7. 215   8. 50,000   9. 4.5   10. 0.15

Rounding off decimals

In clinical veterinary medicine, we do not usually need to measure things to one thousandths or lower, so we can round off our decimals to the nearest hundredth or even the nearest tenth. To do this, we look at the number to the right of the place to which we are rounding. If the number is 5 or greater, we bump up the last number by 1. If it is less than 5, the last number stays the same.

10.56 rounded to the nearest tenth becomes 10.6

10.54 rounded to the nearest tenth becomes 10.5

10.556 rounded to the nearest hundredth becomes 10.56

Remember to look to the number that is one past the rounding point; if rounding to the tenths, look at the number in the hundredths spot.

Converting common fractions to decimals

A fraction can be converted into a decimal by simply dividing the numerator by the denominator. Remember to keep the zero to the left of the decimal point when converting proper fractions.

$$\frac{4}{10} = 4 \div 10 = 0.4, \quad \frac{4}{16} = 4 \div 16 = 0.25,$$

$$\frac{25}{200} = 25 \div 200 = 0.125$$

 Remember to turn mixed numbers into improper fractions before converting them into decimals.

$$12\frac{1}{4} = \frac{49}{4} = 49 \div 4 = 12.25$$

$$7\frac{8}{9} = \frac{71}{9} = 71 \div 9 = 7.89 \text{ (rounded to nearest one hundredth)}$$

Converting decimals into fractions

This conversion is quite simple as we just need to remove the decimal point to give us the numerator and count the number of decimal places in the original number to find our denominator. Simplify the fraction if possible.

$$0.25 = \frac{25}{100} = \frac{1}{4}, \quad 0.005 = \frac{5}{1000} = \frac{1}{200}$$

Decimals greater than 1 are converted to a mixed number by treating the part of the number less than 1 as a proper fraction.

$$5.75 = 5\frac{75}{100} = 5\frac{3}{4}$$

Let's do it again!

Convert the following fractions into decimals and decimals into fractions.

1. $\frac{12}{16}$　2. $\frac{25}{500}$　3. 0.005　4. 52.4　5. 2.025

ANSWERS

1. 0.75　2. 0.05　3. $\frac{1}{200}$　4. $52\frac{2}{5}$　5. $2\frac{1}{40}$

Working with percentages

Percentages are used often in veterinary medicine. We may use 0.9% saline solution for intravenous use, 1% propofol for anaesthesia induction, and a pulse oximeter to determine oxygen saturation as a percentage of the blood oxygen carrying capacity.

Think of the word *percent*; it literally means *per one hundred* (*cent* is one hundred in French). The expression 84% means '84 parts per one hundred parts'. We can express this as a decimal by dropping the percent sign and divide by 100 or 0.01. When we do this, 84% becomes $\frac{84}{100}$ or 0.84. Going the other way, 0.34 becomes 34% and $\frac{2}{10}$ becomes 20% ($\frac{2}{10} = \frac{20}{100}$). Remember to reduce the fractions after converting from a percent. In the examples above, $\frac{84}{100}$ can be reduced to $\frac{21}{25}$ and $\frac{2}{10}$ becomes $\frac{1}{5}$.

We can convert fractions to percentages by converting them into a decimal fraction and then multiplying by 100:

- Divide the numerator by the denominator
- Multiply by 100.

$$\frac{3}{5} = 3 \div 5 = 0.6 \longrightarrow 0.6 \times 100 = 60\%$$

$$\frac{14}{25} = 14 \div 25 = 0.56 \longrightarrow 0.56 \times 100 = 56\%$$

$$4\frac{3}{5} = \frac{23}{5} = 23 \div 5 = 4.6 \longrightarrow 4.6 \times 100 = 460\%$$

Adding and subtracting percentages

Since all percentages are fractions with a denominator of 100, they can be added and subtracted without any other manipulations. For instance, 23% + 10% = 33%. Let's convince ourselves:

$$23\% = \frac{23}{100}, \ 10\% = \frac{10}{100}, \ \frac{23}{100} + \frac{10}{100} = \frac{33}{100} = 33\%$$

 ## Let's do it again!

1. 14% + 2%   2. 45% − 22%   3. 10.5% + 20.4%
4. 67.8% − 22.5%   5. 50% − 0.5%

ANSWERS

1. 16%   2. 23%   3. 30.9%   4. 45.3%   5. 49.5%

Multiplying percentages

We can take any number and multiply it by a percent, or we can take a percent and multiply it by another percent. If I asked: 'What is 3 times 25%?' you would simply multiply 25 by 3 and reply '75%'. If I asked: 'What is 30% of 25%?' you would have a little more work on your hands! You should change one of the percentages to a decimal or a common fraction and then carry out the calculation:

$$30\% = 0.3, \quad 0.3 \times 25\% = 7.5\%$$
$$30\% = \frac{30}{100}, \quad \frac{30}{100} \times 25\% = \frac{750}{100}\% = 7.5\%$$

Let's do it again!

Multiply the following.

1. 67% × 0.5%   2. 20% × 50%   3. 1% × 75%
4. 100% × 20%   5. 0.5% × 25%

ANSWERS

1. 0.335%   2. 10%   3. 0.75%   4. 20%   5. 0.125%

Dividing percentages

The same technique can be applied to division of percentages. If the question involves more than one percentage, simply convert one percentage into a decimal or fraction then carry out the operation:

$$25\% \div 5 = 5\%$$

$$20\% \div 10\% = 20\% \div 0.1 = 200\% \left(\text{or } 20\% \div \frac{1}{10} = 20\% \times \frac{10}{1} = 200\% \right)$$

Making life simpler

If dividing one percentage by another, you can put them in the form of a fraction and cancel the percentages.

$$5\% \div 10\% \longrightarrow \frac{5\%}{10\%} \longrightarrow \frac{5}{10} = \frac{1}{2} = 50\%$$

Let's do it again!

Divide the following.

1. $48\% \div 2$ 2. $\frac{66\%}{3}$ 3. $25\% \div 5\%$ 4. $10\% \div 0.1\%$ 5. $\frac{50\%}{10\%}$

ANSWERS

1. 24% 2. 22% 3. 500% 4. $10,000\%$ 5. 500%

What is scientific notation?

Scientific notation is just a way of expressing very large or very small numbers in a simple form that makes it easier to perform calculations. One application of this concept is in haematology (the study of blood) when the number of red or white cells in a sample is calculated (see Chapter 3). To express a number in scientific notation, we make it a multiple of 10. For example, the number 100 can be expressed as $1 \times 10 \times 10$ or 1×10^2. The number 10,000 can be broken down to $1 \times 10 \times 10 \times 10 \times 10$ or 1×10^4. When using multiples of 10, we call 10 the *base* and the number of times it is multiplied by itself the *exponent*. In 1×10^2, the exponent is 2 and in 1×10^4, the exponent is 4.

 ## Let's do it again!

Express the following numbers in scientific notation.

1. 1000   2. 100,000   3. 1,000,000   4. 10   5. 10,000,000

ANSWERS

1. 1×10^3 2. 1×10^5 3. 1×10^6 4. 1×10^1 5. 1×10^7

Any number can be expressed in this way. Consider 159. How can we express this as a multiple of 10? We move the decimal point to the left until only one digit remains to the left. The exponent of the base 10 is equal to the number of places moved:

$$159 \longrightarrow 1.59 \times 10^2$$

Here are some more examples:

$$1245 \longrightarrow 1.245 \times 10^3$$

$$45{,}678 \longrightarrow 4.5678 \times 10^4$$

$$630{,}000 \longrightarrow 6.3 \times 10^5$$

Numbers smaller than zero can also be expressed in scientific notation, but the exponent will be *negative*. The number 0.1 can be written as 1×10^{-1}. Using a negative exponent means the number is multiplied by a fraction with a denominator that has a base of 10. In other words, 10^{-1} also means $\frac{1}{10}$. The number 0.001 can be written as 1×10^{-3} or as $1 \times \frac{1}{1000}$ or as $1 \times \frac{1}{10} \times \frac{1}{10} \times \frac{1}{10}$.

Any number smaller than 1 can be expressed in scientific notation by moving the decimal point to the right so that one digit remains to the left of the decimal. The exponent is a negative number equal to the number of places moved. Here are some examples:

$$0.012 \longrightarrow 1.2 \times 10^{-2}$$

$$0.00365 \longrightarrow 3.65 \times 10^{-3}$$

$$0.000843 \longrightarrow 8.43 \times 10^{-4}$$

 Let's do it again!

Express each number in scientific notation.
1. 0.14   2. 0.002854   3. 1765   4. 0.0000023   5. 0.000385

ANSWERS

1. 1.4×10^{-1} 2. 2.854×10^{-3} 3. 1.765×10^3
4. 2.3×10^{-6} 5. 3.85×10^{-4}

Barking up the wrong tree

Be careful when working with numbers expressed in scientific notation. Those with negative exponents can fool you! Look at the number 1.345×10^{-4}. This really means $1.345 \times \frac{1}{10,000}$ or, expressed another way, $\frac{1.345}{10,000}$. It does *not* mean $\frac{1}{13,450}$.

Multiplying with scientific notation

When multiplying two numbers expressed in scientific notation, just multiply the numbers and add the exponents to give you the final number:

$(3 \times 10^3) \times (5 \times 10^2) = 15 \times 10^5$ or, more properly expressed, 1.5×10^6 (Move the decimal point until just one number appears to the left of the decimal point and add the equivalent number of spaces moved to the exponent.)

Here are some more examples:

$2 + 4 = 6$

$(2.5 \times 10^2) \times (1.5 \times 10^4) = 3.75 \times 10^6$

$2.5 \times 1.5 = 3.75$

$(3 \times 10^5) \times (2 \times 10^{-3}) = 6 \times 10^2$

$(2 \times 10^{-3}) \times (4 \times 10^{-2}) = 8 \times 10^{-5}$

Let's do it again!

1. $(1 \times 10^6) \times (4 \times 10^5)$ 2. $(2.3 \times 10^{-2}) \times (1.4 \times 10^6)$
3. $(6 \times 10^3) \times (2.2 \times 10^{-9})$

ANSWERS

1. 4×10^{11} 2. 3.22×10^4 3. 1.32×10^{-5}

Dividing with scientific notation

As you might expect, when dividing numbers with scientific notation, we carry out the operation on the numbers that appear before the base 10 and then *subtract* the exponents. Be sure to subtract the exponent of the divisor from the exponent of the dividend. Here are some examples:

$$(2 \times 10^3) \div (1 \times 10^2) = 2 \times 10^1$$

$3 - 2 = 1$

$2 \div 1 = 2$

Dividend

Divisor

$$(8 \times 10^7) \div (2 \times 10^4) = 4 \times 10^3$$
$$(6.6 \times 10^4) \div (2 \times 10^{-2}) = 3.3 \times 10^6$$

 ## Let's do it again!

1. $(2.4 \times 10^{-4}) \div (1.2 \times 10^{-2})$ 2. $\frac{2 \times 10^6}{1 \times 10^3}$
3. $(4.8 \times 10^6) \div (2 \times 10^7)$

ANSWERS

1. 2×10^{-2} 2. 2×10^3 3. 2.4×10^{-1}

Adding and subtracting with scientific notation

When multiplying and dividing, we were able to carry out these operations between two numbers that had different values for the exponents. When adding and subtracting however, we must convert the numbers so that the exponents have the *same value*. After adding the significant figures, the exponent used is the same as that which appears in the two numbers. Here is an example:

Add: $(1 \times 10^5) + (3 \times 10^4)$

Step 1: $1 \times 10^5 \longrightarrow 10 \times 10^4$

Step 2: $(10 \times 10^4) + (3 \times 10^4) = 13 \times 10^4$ or 1.3×10^5

Note that we could have changed the other exponent:

$3 \times 10^4 \longrightarrow 0.3 \times 10^5$

$(1 \times 10^5) + (0.3 \times 10^5) = 1.3 \times 10^5$

 ## Making life simpler

If in doubt when performing operations involving scientific notation, change the number to its regular form and carry on. For example:

$(5 \times 10^4) - (3 \times 10^3)$ becomes

$50,000 - 3000 = 47000 = 4.7 \times 10^4$

 ## Let's do it again!

1. $(4.3 \times 10^5) + (2.1 \times 10^2)$ 2. $(6.75 \times 10^{-2}) - (2.6 \times 10^{-4})$
3. $(1.25 \times 10^3) + (4.25 \times 10^2)$

ANSWERS

1. 4.3021×10^5 2. 6.724×10^{-2} 3. 1.675×10^3

Multiple choice questions

1. $6\frac{3}{8}$ is the same as which improper fraction?

   a. $\frac{24}{8}$ b. $\frac{51}{4}$ c. $\frac{48}{8}$ d. $\frac{51}{8}$

2. $4\frac{4}{7}$ is the same as which of the following?

   a. $\frac{24}{7}$ b. $\frac{16}{7}$ c. $\frac{8}{7}$ d. $\frac{32}{7}$

3. $2\frac{5}{9}$ is the same as which of the following fractions?

   a. $\frac{23}{3}$ b. $\frac{23}{9}$ c. $\frac{10}{9}$ d. $\frac{18}{3}$

4. $3\frac{3}{10}$ is equal to

   a. $\frac{33}{10}$ b. $\frac{30}{10}$ c. $\frac{9}{10}$ d. $\frac{57}{5}$

5. $\frac{54}{7}$ is equal to

   a. $4\frac{5}{7}$ b. $6\frac{5}{7}$ c. $7\frac{5}{7}$ d. $7\frac{4}{7}$

Answers

1. d. $\frac{51}{8}$

2. d. $\frac{32}{7}$

3. b. $\frac{23}{9}$

4. a. $\frac{33}{10}$

5. c. $7\frac{5}{7}$

Chapter 2

Methods of solving for the unknown

Learning Objectives

- What is a ratio?
- What is a proportion?
- Solving for x
- What is dimensional analysis?
- How to identify conversion factors
- How to set up an equation using dimensional analysis

Ratio and proportion

What is a ratio?

A ratio is a way of demonstrating the *relationship between two numbers*. Ratios are used extensively in veterinary medicine. Think of an antibiotic tablet that is labelled as 100 mg. This implies that one tablet contains 100 mg of active ingredient, and can be expressed as:

1 tablet:100 mg or 100 mg:1 tablet

We can also express this relationship as a fraction:

$$\frac{1 \text{ tablet}}{100 \text{ mg}} \quad \text{or} \quad \frac{100 \text{ mg}}{1 \text{ tablet}}$$

The concentration of liquid medication is often expressed as a ratio. The anaesthetic propofol comes in a concentration of 10 mg per millilitre (mL) and would appear as 10 mg/mL (10 mg per 1 mL).

What is a proportion?

A proportion demonstrates the *relationship between two ratios*. In a true proportion, the two ratios are equal. Using the 100 mg tablets, we can say if one tablet contains 100 mg, then two tablets contain 200 mg. We can express this:

$$1 \text{ tablet}:100 \text{ mg} = 2 \text{ tablets}:200 \text{ mg} \quad \text{or} \quad \frac{1 \text{ tablet}}{100 \text{ mg}} = \frac{2 \text{ tablets}}{200 \text{ mg}}$$

The fraction method is more commonly used to express ratios and proportions, so we will use this from now on.

When setting up a ratio and proportion statement, we must ensure the order of the ratio on one side of the equal sign is the same as on the other side. In the statement above, tablets are on top of ratios and mg are on the bottom. We cannot put tablets on top on one side and on the bottom on the other and expect both sides of the equation to be equal:

$$\frac{1 \text{ tablet}}{100 \text{ mg}} \neq \frac{200 \text{ mg}}{2 \text{ tablets}}$$

Remember to pay close attention to the equal sign. One side of the equation must equal the other side. Think of $\frac{1}{2}$ and $\frac{2}{4}$ – the numbers are different, but the value is the same.

Using ratio and proportion to solve for *x*

Since one side of a ratio and proportion statement must equal the other side, if three values of the statement are supplied, we can use the relationship to determine the fourth value. Consider the question: 'If each tablet contains 100 mg, how many mg do two tablets contain?'

We set up the ratio and proportion statement:

$$\frac{1 \text{ tablet}}{100 \text{ mg}} = \frac{2 \text{ tablets}}{x \text{ mg}}$$

In a true proportion, the products of cross multiplication are equal therefore:

1 tablet   2 tablets

100 mg   x mg

(1 tablet) $(x\text{ mg})$ = (2 tablets) (100 mg)

Recall from your early days of mathematics that whatever we do to one side of the equation, we can also do to the other side and not change the relationship. In the equation above, we can divide both sides by one tablet:

$$\frac{(1 \text{ tablet})(x \text{ mg})}{1 \text{ tablet}} = \frac{(2 \text{ tablets})(100 \text{ mg})}{1 \text{ tablet}}$$

We can also cancel units that appear in the numerator and denominator:

$$\frac{(1 \ \cancel{\text{tablet}})(x \text{ mg})}{1 \ \cancel{\text{tablet}}} = \frac{(2 \ \cancel{\text{tablets}})(100 \text{ mg})}{1 \ \cancel{\text{tablet}}}$$

$$x \text{ mg} = (2)(100 \text{ mg})$$
$$x = 200 \text{ mg}$$

Dimensional analysis

What is dimensional analysis?

Dimensional analysis sounds very technical but it is actually a very simple and logical method of converting units of measurement from one form to another. In chemistry courses, you may have used this method under the name *factor label method or unit factor method*. In the medical sciences, we often face problems where we are dealing with different types of measurement, and this method allows us to change the measurement type to fit the situation.

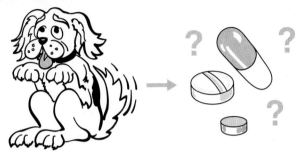

Fig. 2.1 Tablet strength and patient size are interrelated

Consider giving a dog an antibiotic tablet. Somehow we have to convert the size of the dog to an equivalent size of tablet (Fig. 2.1) based on a dosage. The first piece of information we need is the weight of the dog – we call this the *starting factor*. It is the unit of measurement that has to be converted to another unit. Second, we need to identify the units of measurement we wish to end up using – we call this the *answer unit*. In this case it is the number of tablets to give to the dog.

How do we arrive at the answer unit from the starting factor? We use one or a series of *conversion factors*. Conversion factors are ratios of units of measurement that have a true relationship and are expressed as fractions with a numerator and denominator. An example of a conversion factor is 3 feet = 1 yard. As a ratio we would show this as:

$$\frac{3 \text{ feet}}{1 \text{ yard}}$$

Another example is: 'There are 1000 mg in 1 g':

$$\frac{1000 \text{ mg}}{1 \text{ g}}$$

Let's go back to our example of a dog requiring an antibiotic tablet. If our dog weighs 10 kg, we use this as our starting factor. The answer unit will be the number of tablets:

Weight (kg) $\longrightarrow$ No. of tablets

To get from our starting factor to our answer unit, we need to multiply the starting factor by one or more conversion factors that serve as *bridges*. The first bridge we need is the dosage – in this case, the amount of antibiotic needed to be effective is 10 mg of antibiotic for every kg the dog weighs:

$$\frac{10 \text{ mg}}{1 \text{ kg}}$$

The second bridge is the amount of antibiotic in each tablet – in this case, each tablet contains 50 mg of antibiotic:

$$\frac{1 \text{ tablet}}{50 \text{ mg}}$$

Let's insert our bridges (conversion factors) in order to arrive at our destination:

$$10 \text{ kg} \times \frac{10 \text{ mg}}{1 \text{ kg}} \times \frac{1 \text{ tablet}}{50 \text{ mg}} = x \text{ tablets}$$

 Remember we can simplify fractions and cancel out units that appear in the numerator and denominator.

So our equation becomes:

Starting factor

$$10 \text{ kg} \times \frac{10 \text{ mg}}{1 \text{ kg}} \times \frac{1 \text{ tablet}}{50 \text{ mg}} = \frac{100 \text{ tablets}}{50} = 2 \text{ tablets}$$

Conversion factors

Answer unit

When setting up your equation, remember to ensure your answer unit is on the top of the conversion factor. In the example above, tablets are the numerator (top) of the conversion factor and mg is denominator (bottom) so that the answer comes out in number of tablets, which is what we are looking for (answer unit).

Dimensional analysis allows us to perform operations without memorizing formulas and allows us to simplify equations so that a calculator is often unnecessary! It can be used in all sorts of situations involving measurements – not just in the clinic.

 Many people were raised with and taught one system of measurement and then in later life faced the introduction of new systems. Dimensional analysis can allow us to convert from one to the other effortlessly (okay, with maybe just a little effort!).

While dimensional analysis is very useful in the clinic, it is also handy to solve every day problems, for instance, if I fill up my car with 40 L of gasoline after having driven 400 km, how efficient is my car expressed in miles per (imperial) gallon?

Starting factor: $\dfrac{\text{kilometres (km)}}{\text{litre (L)}}$ Answer unit: $\dfrac{\text{miles}}{\text{gallon}}$

Conversion factors: 1 gallon = 4.55 L   8 km = 5 miles

$$\frac{400 \text{ km}}{40 \text{ L}} \times \frac{4.55 \text{ L}}{1 \text{ gallon}} \times \frac{5 \text{ miles}}{8 \text{ km}} = \frac{9100 \text{ miles}}{320 \text{ gallons}} = \frac{28.4 \text{ miles}}{1 \text{ gallon}}$$

Identifying conversion factors

Conversion factors have values that are relative to each other. In other words, they represent a *ratio*. The relative value has to be true – you can't just make something up! Some standard conversion factors are:

12 inches   =   1 foot

1000 millimetre   =   1 metre

60 seconds   =   1 minute

Other conversion factors are determined by the nature of the problem. If tablets come in 100 mg strength, then the conversion factor is 1 tablet = 100 mg. If the rate of fluid administration is supposed to be set at 10 mL per hour, then the conversion factor is 10 mL = 1 hour.

The key is the relative value. Whether I give one tablet or 100 mg, as in the example above, I am giving the same amount. In the last example, with the passage of 1 hour, 10 mL will have been administered (conversely, if 10 mL has been administered, then 1 hour must have passed). Since the two values are relative, multiplying the starting factor by the conversion factor does not change the value of the starting factor but does change the way it looks. Thus, we can convert a 10-kg dog into two 50-mg tablets!

Setting up the equation

Setting up an equation using dimensional analysis can be broken down into these seven steps:

1. Identify the starting factor
2. Identify the answer units
3. Determine the conversion factors needed
4. Ensure the conversion factors are in the correct format to give you the desired answer unit
5. Cancel units that appear in both the numerator and denominator
6. Simplify the fractions
7. Complete the equation.

 Barking up the wrong tree

When using conversion factors, it is very important to consider what to place in the numerator and what to place in the denominator. For instance, if we say each tablet is 100 mg, we can either express this as:

$$\frac{1\ \text{tablet}}{100\ \text{mg}} \quad \text{or} \quad \frac{100\ \text{mg}}{1\ \text{tablet}}$$

How do we decide how to express the ratio? We always leave the units we want to end up with *on top*. If we are determining how many tablets to give, we use:

$$\frac{1\ \text{tablet}}{100\ \text{mg}}$$

If we are trying to determine how many mg to give, we use:

$$\frac{100 \text{ mg}}{1 \text{ tablet}}$$

Be sure to put your conversion factors in the correct format to give you the required answer unit.

Let's do it again!

Determine the value of x in the following proportions.

1. $\frac{75 \text{ mg}}{5 \text{ mL}} = \frac{187.5 \text{ mg}}{x \text{ mL}}$ 2. $\frac{17 \text{ mg}}{3 \text{ tabs}} = \frac{42.5 \text{ mg}}{x \text{ tabs}}$ 3. $\frac{55 \text{ mg}}{1.1 \text{ mL}} = \frac{165 \text{ mg}}{x \text{ mL}}$

4. $\frac{250 \text{ U}}{2.5 \text{ mL}} = \frac{30 \text{ U}}{x \text{ mL}}$ 5. $\frac{12.5 \text{ mg}}{1.2 \text{ mL}} = \frac{6.25 \text{ mg}}{x \text{ mL}}$

ANSWERS

1. $x = 12.5$ mL   2. 7.5 tabs   3. 3.3 mL   4. 0.3 mL

5. 0.6 mL

Let's do it again!

Use dimensional analysis to solve the following problems.

1. A 5-kg cat requires $\frac{25 \text{ mg}}{\text{kg}}$ of medication that comes in a liquid strength of $\frac{10 \text{ mg}}{1 \text{ mL}}$. How many mL of liquid medication are you to give?
2. A 33-lb dog needs 100 mg/kg of medication that comes in tablets of 500 mg. How many tablets do you give?

ANSWERS

1. $5 \text{ kg} \times \dfrac{25 \text{ mg}}{\text{kg}} \times \dfrac{1 \text{ mL}}{10 \text{ mg}} = 12.5 \text{ mL}$

2. $33 \text{ lb} \times \dfrac{1 \text{ kg}}{2.2 \text{ lb}} \times \dfrac{100 \text{ mg}}{\text{kg}} \times \dfrac{1 \text{ tablet}}{500 \text{ mg}} = 3 \text{ tablets}$

Multiple choice questions

1. $\dfrac{52}{8} = \dfrac{312}{x}$

   a. 6   b. 40   c. 48   d. 88

2. $\dfrac{6.4}{4} = \dfrac{3.2}{x}$

   a. 1   b. 2   c. 3.2   d. 6.4

3. $\dfrac{23.24}{3.8} = \dfrac{97.61}{x}$

   a. 3.8   b. 4.2   c. 5.96   d. 15.96

4. $\dfrac{8}{1} = \dfrac{38.4}{x}$

   a. 1   b. 2.4   c. 4.8   d. 8

5. $\dfrac{136}{36} = \dfrac{19.43}{x}$

   a. 5.14   b. 14.5   c. 15.4   d. 51.4

Answers

1. c. 48
2. b. 2
3. d. 15.96
4. c. 4.8
5. a. 5.14

Chapter 3

Clinical applications of basic principles

Let's see how everyday problems in a typical small animal practice can be solved using the concepts we have reviewed. When solving word problems that mimic those you will find in real life, always ask yourself a few questions to help organize your work. What value am I trying to find? It could be the number of tablets to give, the amount of fluids to administer, or the percentage of weight loss a dog needs to be healthy. Then ask yourself what information is provided and is it all relevant? This could be the strength of the tablets, the degree of dehydration of the patient or the current weight of a dog. Set up your work by devising how to take the information provided in order to end up with the answer you are seeking and determine what method will suit the problem. Answers begin on page 38.

Questions

1. You must give a dog 250 mg of a medication that comes in tablets labelled 100 mg each. How many tablets will you give?
2. A dog weighs 60 kg and you tell the owner his dog should only weigh 50 kg. What fraction of its current weight must it lose to achieve the goal weight?
3. For the dog in question 2, what percent of its current weight (to the nearest tenth) does this represent?

4. A cat requires 50 mg of a liquid medication that has a strength of 150 mg/mL. What fraction of a mL should be given?

5. A dog on intravenous fluids has received 30% of the 500 mL initially in the i.v. bag. How many mL has it received?

6. If the dog in the question above weighs 25 kg, how many mL per kg of body weight has it received?

7. Tablets are 300 micrograms (μg) each and you must give 125 μg. What fraction of a tablet will you give?

8. A cat is to receive 90 kcal of a canned food at each meal. The food has a caloric density of 360 kcal per can. What fraction of a can should it receive at each meal?

9. A blood sample is diluted by placing 0.1 mL of the blood in a tube and filling the tube to the 20-mL mark with a solution. What percent of the solution represents whole blood?

10. Tablet A has a strength of 0.125 mg and tablet B has a strength of $\frac{1}{7}$ mg. Which tablet is stronger?

11. A clinic has 5250 patients of which 2020 are dogs, 2580 are cats, 400 are 'pocket pets' and the rest are birds. Determine the percentage of each category (answer to the nearest tenth).

12. If the same distribution in question 11 held true with 10,000 patients, how many pets would be in each category?

13. A dog ate $\frac{2}{3}$ of a cup of dry food in the morning, $\frac{1}{4}$ of a cup in the afternoon and $\frac{1}{2}$ of a cup in the evening. If the food has a caloric density of 350 kcal per cup, how many kcal did the dog eat in total (answer to nearest tenth)?

14. A cat that swallowed a string needs to have surgery to remove part of its small intestine. If 15 cm is removed and the total length of the small intestine was 300 cm, what percent of intestine did the cat lose?

15. A volume of 15 mL of an anaesthetic drug was drawn into a syringe. Initially, $\frac{1}{3}$ was injected followed by $\frac{1}{2}$ of the remainder. What fraction of the total drawn up did the patient receive?

16. When performing a complete blood count on a dog, you determine the leukocyte (white blood cell) total to be 5×10^3

cells/μL. If there are 1×10^6 μL in every L, what was the count in cell per L? Hint: Set it up as a ratio and proportion:

$$\frac{5 \times 10^3 \text{ cells}}{1\ \mu L} = \frac{x \text{ cells}}{1 \times 10^6\ \mu L}$$

Use ratio and proportion equations to solve the following

17. A 5-kg cat needs amoxicillin at 22 mg/kg. How many mg of amoxicillin will you give?
18. A 45-kg dog needs prednisolone at 2.2 mg/kg. How many mg of prednisolone will you give?
19. A 20-kg dog needs 30 mg/kg of a medication that comes in 300-mg tablets. How many tablets will you give?
20. A 4-kg cat requires a liquid medication at 15 mg/kg. The liquid comes in a strength of 100 mg/mL. How many mL will you give?
21. An American family visiting London with their dog requires veterinary services that cost 356 GBP. Each US dollar is equivalent to 0.74 GB pounds. How much is their bill in US dollars?

Use dimensional analysis to solve the following

22. A 5-kg cat needs an antibiotic at a dose of 15 mg/kg. The antibiotic comes in liquid form at a concentration of 125 mg/5 mL. How many mL do you give?
23. A cat weighing 4.5 kg needs insulin at 1.5 international units (IU) per kg. The insulin comes in a strength of 10 IU/mL. How much insulin do you give (answer to nearest tenth of a mL)?
24. What volume of fluid does a patient receive in 6 hours with a fluid rate of 30 mL/h?

Answers

1. $$\frac{100 \text{ mg}}{1 \text{ tablet}} = \frac{250 \text{ mg}}{x \text{ tablets}}$$

   $(250 \text{ mg})(1 \text{ tab}) = (100 \text{ mg})(x \text{ tabs})$

   $$x \text{ tabs} = \frac{250 \text{ mg}}{100 \text{ mg}} = 2.5 \text{ tabs}$$

2. 60 kg current weight – 50 kg goal weight = 10 kg weight loss

   $$\frac{10 \text{ kg}}{60 \text{ kg}} = \frac{1}{6}$$

3. $\frac{1}{6} = 0.167, \quad 0.167 \times 100 = 16.7\%$

4. $\frac{150 \text{ mg}}{1 \text{ mL}} = \frac{50 \text{ mg}}{x \text{ mL}}, \quad (150 \text{ mg})(x \text{ mL}) = (50 \text{ mg})(1 \text{ mL})$

   $$x \text{ mL} = \frac{(50 \text{ mg})(1 \text{ mL})}{150 \text{ mg}}, \quad x = \frac{1}{3}\text{mL}$$

5. $500 \text{ mL} \times 30\% = 500 \text{ mL} \times 0.3 \left(\frac{30}{100}\right) = 150 \text{ mL}$

   $\frac{30}{100} = 0.3 = 30\%$

6. $\frac{150 \text{ mL}}{25 \text{ kg}} = \frac{x \text{ mL}}{1 \text{ kg}}$

   $(150 \text{ mL})(1 \text{ kg}) = (x \text{ mL})(25 \text{ kg})$

   $$x \text{ mL} = \frac{(150 \text{ mL})(1 \text{ kg})}{25 \text{ kg}} = 6 \text{ mL}$$

7. $\frac{125 \text{ µg}}{300 \text{ µg}} = \frac{5}{12}$

8. $\dfrac{90 \text{ kcal}}{360 \text{ kcal}} = \dfrac{1}{4}$

9. $\dfrac{0.1 \text{ mL}}{20 \text{ mL}} = 0.005, \quad 0.005 \times 100 = 0.5\%$

10. $0.125 \text{ mg} = \dfrac{125}{1000} = \dfrac{1}{8} \text{ mg}$

$\dfrac{1}{7} \text{ mg} > \dfrac{1}{8} \text{ mg}$

11. $\dfrac{2020}{5250} = 0.3847, \quad 0.385 \times 100 = 38.5\%$ are dogs

$\dfrac{2580}{5250} = 0.4914, \quad 0.491 \times 100 = 49.1\%$ are cats

$\dfrac{400}{5250} = 0.0761, \quad 0.076 \times 100 = 7.6\%$ are 'pocket pets'

$\dfrac{5250 - (2020 + 2580 + 400)}{5250} = 0.0476$

$0.0480 \times 100 = 4.8\%$ are birds

12. $38.5\% \text{ dogs} \times 10{,}000 \text{ patients} = 0.385 \times 10{,}000 = 3850 \text{ dogs}$

$49.1\% \text{ cats} \times 10{,}000 \text{ patients} = 0.491 \times 10{,}000 = 4910 \text{ cats}$

$7.6\% \text{ pocket pets} \times 10{,}000 \text{ patients} = 0.076 \times 10{,}000$
$$= 760 \text{ pocket pets}$$

$4.8\% \text{ birds} \times 10{,}000 \text{ patients} = 0.048 \times 10{,}000 = 480 \text{ birds}$

13. $\dfrac{2}{3} + \dfrac{1}{4} + \dfrac{1}{2} = \dfrac{8}{12} + \dfrac{3}{12} + \dfrac{6}{12} = \dfrac{17}{12}$

$\dfrac{17}{12} \text{ cup} \times \dfrac{350 \text{ kcal}}{\text{cup}} = 495.8 \text{ kcal}$

14. $\dfrac{15 \text{ cm}}{300 \text{ cm}} = 0.05, \quad 0.05 \times 100 = 5\%$

15. $\dfrac{1}{3} \times 15 \text{ mL} = 5 \text{ mL}, \quad \dfrac{1}{2} \times (15 \text{ mL} - 5 \text{ mL}) = 5 \text{ mL}$

$\dfrac{(5 \text{ mL} + 5 \text{ mL})}{15 \text{ mL}} = \dfrac{2}{3}$

16. $\dfrac{5 \times 10^3 \text{ cells}}{1 \text{ } \mu\text{L}} = \dfrac{x \text{ cells}}{1 \times 10^6 \text{ } \mu\text{L}}$

$(x \text{ cells})(1 \text{ } \mu\text{L}) = (5 \times 10^3 \text{ cells})(1 \times 10^6 \text{ } \mu\text{L})$

$x = 5 \times 10^9 \text{ cells/L}$

17. $\dfrac{22 \text{ mg}}{1 \text{ kg}} = \dfrac{x \text{ mg}}{5 \text{ kg}}, \quad (22 \text{ mg})(5 \text{ kg}) = (x \text{ mg})(1 \text{ kg})$

$x \text{ mg} = \dfrac{(22 \text{ mg})(5 \text{ kg})}{1 \text{ kg}} = 110 \text{ mg}$

18. $\dfrac{2.2 \text{ mg}}{1 \text{ kg}} = \dfrac{x \text{ mg}}{45 \text{ kg}}, \quad (2.2 \text{ mg})(45 \text{ kg}) = (x \text{ mg})(1 \text{ kg})$

$x \text{ mg} = \dfrac{(2.2 \text{ mg})(45 \text{ kg})}{1 \text{ kg}} = 99 \text{ mg}$

19. $\dfrac{30 \text{ mg}}{1 \text{ kg}} = \dfrac{x \text{ mg}}{20 \text{ kg}}, \quad (30 \text{ mg})(20 \text{ kg}) = (x \text{ mg})(1 \text{ kg}), \quad x = 600 \text{ mg}$

$\dfrac{300 \text{ mg}}{1 \text{ tab}} = \dfrac{600 \text{ mg}}{x \text{ tabs}}$

$(600 \text{ mg})(1 \text{ tab}) = (300 \text{ mg})(x \text{ tabs}), \quad x = 2 \text{ tabs}$

20. $\dfrac{15 \text{ mg}}{1 \text{ kg}} = \dfrac{x \text{ mg}}{4 \text{ kg}}, \quad x = 60 \text{ mg}$

$\dfrac{100 \text{ mg}}{1 \text{ mL}} = \dfrac{60 \text{ mg}}{x \text{ mL}}, \quad (60 \text{ mg})(1 \text{ mL}) = (100 \text{ mg})(x \text{ mL}), x = 0.6 \text{ mL}$

21. $\dfrac{1\ \text{USD}}{0.74\ \text{GBP}} = \dfrac{x\ \text{USD}}{356\ \text{GBP}}$

$x = 481.08$ USD

22. Starting factor: 5 kg (weight of cat)

Answer unit: Number of mL

Conversion factors: $\dfrac{15\ \text{mg}}{1\ \text{kg}}$ (dosage), $\dfrac{5\ \text{mL}}{125\ \text{mg}}$

(strength of antibiotic)

$5\ \cancel{\text{kg}} \times \dfrac{15\ \cancel{\text{mg}}}{1\ \cancel{\text{kg}}} \times \dfrac{5\ \text{mL}}{125\ \cancel{\text{mg}}} = 3\ \text{mL}$

23. Starting factor: 4.5 kg (weight of cat)

Answer unit: Number of mL

Conversion factors: $\dfrac{1.5\ \text{IU}}{1\ \text{kg}}$ (dosage), $\dfrac{1\ \text{mL}}{10\ \text{IU}}$

(strength of insulin)

$4.5\ \cancel{\text{kg}} \times \dfrac{1.5\ \cancel{\text{IU}}}{1\ \cancel{\text{kg}}} \times \dfrac{1\ \text{mL}}{10\ \cancel{\text{IU}}} = 0.7\ \text{mL}$

24. Starting factor: 6 hours

Answer unit: Number of mL of fluid

Conversion factor: $\dfrac{30\ \text{mL}}{1\ \text{h}}$ (fluid rate)

$6\ \cancel{\text{h}} \times \dfrac{30\ \text{mL}}{1\ \cancel{\text{h}}} = 180\ \text{mL}$

Multiple choice questions

1. Your patient requires feeding through a feeding tube. He needs 365 kcal/day divided into six feeds. The liquid feed contains 2.1 kcal/mL. How many mL does he need per feed (round to the nearest mL)?

   a. 29 mL   b. 35 mL   c. 102 mL   d. 127 mL

2. A 15-kg dog requires treatment of cyclosporine 100 mg/mL for atopic dermatitis. The recommended dose is 5 mg/kg once daily for 4 weeks. The vials are available in 5, 15, 30 and 50 mL. Which size bottle would be needed to allow the full course?

   a. 5 mL   b. 15 mL   c. 30 mL   d. 50 mL

3. A dog attends your weight clinic, she currently weighs 27 kg and needs to lose 20% of her bodyweight. What is her target weight to the nearest kg?

   a. 15 kg   b. 22 kg   c. 32 kg   d. 35 kg

4. Tablets are available in 175-mg strength. Your patient requires 60 mg, how much of the tablet do you administer?

   a. One quarter   b. One third
   c. Half   d. Three quarters

5. A dog has been prescribed medication in the form of 80-mg tablets. The patient requires 20 mg. What fraction of the tablet do you administer?

   a. $\frac{1}{2}$ b. $\frac{1}{3}$ c. $\frac{1}{4}$ d. $\frac{1}{5}$

Answers

1. a. 29 mL
2. c. 30 mL
3. b. 22 kg
4. b. One third
5. c. $\frac{1}{4}$

Chapter 4

Measurement systems

Learning Objectives

- Review the metric system
- Convert values within the metric system
- Solve clinical problems using the metric system
- Review other common systems of measure
- Convert values from other systems to the metric system

The metric system

The metric system is the most commonly used system of measure in the world and is used almost exclusively within medical professions. It is based on the decimal system – using a base of 10. This makes calculations and conversions relatively simple.

The three basic things we want to measure are weight, volume and length (Fig. 4.1).

Weight – basic unit is the gram (abbreviated g)

Volume – basic unit is the litre (abbreviated L)

Length – basic unit is the metre (abbreviated m)

Fig. 4.1   Basic units of measurement for common variables

 Worlds apart

In the United States, the preferred spelling of litre is liter and
that of metre is meter. In Canada, both forms are encountered.
Fortunately, the abbreviations are the same!

The basic unit of each measurement can be modified to indicate a larger or smaller quantity. This is accomplished by the
addition of prefixes that carry a specific meaning (Table 4.1).

Converting within the metric system

The beauty of the metric system is its simplicity – we should all
be able to divide or multiply by 10! If we remember the commonly
used units in the table, we can move from one unit to another.

Table 4.1   Prefixes in measurement units. Commonly used units are shown in bold type

Prefix	Symbol	Multiple of base unit	Weight	Volume	Length
Mega	M	1,000,000 (10^6)	Megagram (Mg)	Megalitre (ML)	Megametre (Mm)
Kilo	k	1000 (10^3)	**Kilogram (kg)**	Kilolitre (kL)	Kilometre (km)
Base unit	–	**1**	**Gram (g)**	**Litre (L)**	**Metre (m)**
Deci	d	0.1 (10^{-1})	Decigram (dg)	Decilitre (dL)	Decimetre (dm)
Centi	c	0.01 (10^{-2})	Centigram (cg)	Centilitre (cL)	Centimetre (cm)
Milli	m	0.001 (10^{-3})	**Milligram (mg)**	**Millilitre (mL)**	**Millimetre (mm)**
Micro	μ or mc	0.000001 (10^{-6})	**Microgram (µg)**	**Microlitre (µL)**	**Micrometre (µm)**

Let's say we want to change 1 cm into metres. We can see that 1 cm is 0.01 of a metre, or in other words there are 100 cm in 1 m. Moving from one to another is easily done by making *conversion factors* and employing dimensional analysis:

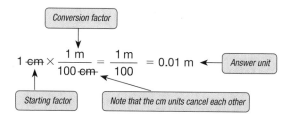

Now I would like to know how many mg are in a 2-g tablet:

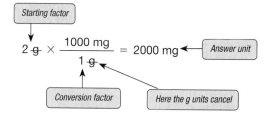

Let's do it again!

1. How many cm are there in 1.8 km?
2. 4 g equals how many µg?
3. How many mL are there in 4.5 L?
4. A mouse weighs 30 g. How would you write this in kg?
5. How many L are there in 100 dL?

ANSWERS

1. $1.8 \, \cancel{km} \times \dfrac{1000 \, \cancel{m}}{1 \, \cancel{km}} \times \dfrac{100 \, cm}{1 \, \cancel{m}} = 180{,}000 \, cm$

2. $4 \, \cancel{g} \times \dfrac{10^6 \, mg}{1 \, \cancel{g}} = 4 \times 10^6 \, mg$

3. $4.5 \, \cancel{L} \times \dfrac{1000 \, mL}{1 \, \cancel{L}} = 4500 \, mL$

4. $30 \, \cancel{g} \times \dfrac{1 \, kg}{1000 \, \cancel{g}} = 0.03 \, kg$

5. $100 \, \cancel{dL} \times \dfrac{1 \, L}{10 \, \cancel{dL}} = 10 \, L$

Clinical applications

There are many problems encountered in veterinary practice that are simplified if you are comfortable moving around in the metric system.

Consider a 20-kg dog that requires 50 mg/kg of a medication that comes in 2-g tablets. How many tablets do we give?

We set the problem up using dimensional analysis:

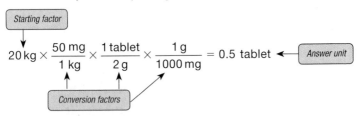

$$20 \, kg \times \dfrac{50 \, mg}{1 \, kg} \times \dfrac{1 \, tablet}{2 \, g} \times \dfrac{1 \, g}{1000 \, mg} = 0.5 \, tablet$$

Starting factor

Answer unit

Conversion factors

Let's take a closer look at the conversion factors:

$$\frac{50 \text{ mg}}{1 \text{ kg}} = \text{dosage}$$

$$\frac{1 \text{ tablet}}{2 \text{ g}} = \text{strength of the medication}$$

$$\frac{1 \text{ g}}{1000 \text{ mg}} = \text{metric conversion factor}$$

Remember to arrange the conversion factors so that all the units except the desired answer units cancel out. In this case, kg, mg and g all appear once in the numerators and once in the denominators, cancelling each other. The only units left are tablets, which is what we want!

Dimensional analysis versus ratio and proportion

Many textbooks will use ratio and proportion to solve dosage calculation problems. This method requires more steps, but for some people it may be preferred. Let's look at the same problem using ratio and proportion:

Step 1: How many mg to give?

$$\frac{50 \text{ mg}}{1 \text{ kg}} = \frac{x \text{ mg}}{20 \text{ kg}}, \quad x = 1000 \text{ mg}$$

Step 2: How many grams does that equal?

$$\frac{1000 \text{ mg}}{1 \text{ g}} = \frac{1000 \text{ mg}}{x \text{ g}}, \quad x = 1 \text{ g}$$

Step 3: How many mg to give?

$$\frac{1 \text{ tablet}}{2 \text{ g}} = \frac{x \text{ tablets}}{1 \text{ g}}, \quad x = 0.5 \text{ tablet}$$

Dimensional analysis allows many steps to be incorporated into one equation, and if set up correctly, once all the cancelling is done, only the desired answer units are left at the end.

Let's do it again!

1. A 30-g mouse requires 200 µg/kg of a medication that only comes in a strength of 1 mg/mL. How many mL do you give?
2. A horse requires intravenous fluids given at a rate of 500 mL/hour. After 7 hours, how many litres will the horse receive?
3. A typical feline ovariohysterectomy (spay operation) requires 5 mL of isoflurane anaesthetic. If a veterinary clinic performs 200 such operations in a month, how many 2-dL bottles of isoflurane will they require?

ANSWERS

1. $30 \text{ g} \times \dfrac{200 \text{ µg}}{1 \text{ kg}} \times \dfrac{1 \text{ kg}}{1000 \text{ g}} \times \dfrac{1 \text{ mL}}{1 \text{ mg}} \times \dfrac{1 \text{ mg}}{1000 \text{ µg}} = 0.006 \text{ mL}$

2. $7 \text{ h} \times \dfrac{500 \text{ mL}}{1 \text{ h}} \times \dfrac{1 \text{ L}}{1000 \text{ mL}} = 3.5 \text{ L}$

3. $200 \text{ ops} \times \dfrac{5 \text{ mL}}{1 \text{ op}} \times \dfrac{1 \text{ bottle}}{2 \text{ dL}} \times \dfrac{1 \text{ dL}}{100 \text{ mL}} = 5 \text{ bottles}$

   (op = operation)

cc: a carbon copy of mL

Although the preferred metric measure for small volumes is millilitre (mL), you may see a drug order given in cubic centimetres (cc). This is because 1 cc of water is equal to 1 mL at a temperature of 4°C (Fig. 4.2).

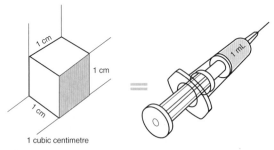

Fig. 4.2 One cubic centimetre is equivalent to one millilitre

Other systems of measure

Household system

Depending on the part of the world in which you live, the household system (Table 4.2) may be more familiar to animal owners than the metric system. This system uses droppers, teaspoons, tablespoons and cups for liquid volume. It is often combined with either the imperial system of measure (in the United Kingdom, Canada, Australia and New Zealand) or the United States Customary System (in the United States). There may be times when you need to direct owners to use this system to administer over-the-counter medications or food supplements.

We can use dimensional analysis to convert within the household system, just as we did within the metric system, using conversion factors from the table below.

Converting between the household and metric system

It may be necessary to convert from one system to another. For instance, if you wanted an owner to administer 5 mL of a liquid anti-diarrhoea preparation to her small dog and she did not have an appropriate metric measuring device, you could tell her how to use a teaspoon measure (1 tsp). Now, it makes a difference where you are in the world as the imperial and US systems are different. Use Table 4.3 for the *approximate* conversions.

Table 4.2 Household systems of measurement	
Household system (US)	**Household system (imperial)**
60 drops (gtt) = 1 teaspoon (tsp)	60 drops (gtt) = 1 teaspoon (tsp)
3 tsp = 1 tablespoon (tbs)	3 tsp = 1 tablespoon (tbs)
2 tbs = 1 ounce (oz)	2 tbs = 1 ounce (oz)
16 oz = 1 pint (pt)	20 oz = 1 pint (pt)
2 pt = 1 quart (qt)	2 pt = 1 quart (qt)
4 qt = 1 gallon (gal)	4 qt = 1 gallon (gal)

Table 4.3 Equivalencies for volume in different measurement systems

Household system	Imperial system metric equivalent	US system metric equivalent
1 tsp	5 mL	5 mL
1 tbs	15 mL	15 mL
1 oz	28 mL	30 mL
1 cup	230 mL	240 mL
1 pint	570 mL	470 mL
1 quart	1.14 L	0.95 L
1 gallon	4.55 L	3.79 L

Table 4.4 Equivalencies for weight and length

Metric	Household system	Household system	Metric system
1 g	0.033 ounce (oz)	1 ounce	30 g
1 kg	2.2 pounds (lb)	1 pound	0.454 kg
1 cm	0.39 inch	1 inch	2.54 cm
		1 foot	30.48 cm
1 m	1.09 yard	1 yard	91.44 cm
1 km	0.625 mile	1 mile	1.6 km

Fortunately, when it comes to weight and length, there is only one set of conversions (Table 4.4).

Let's go through a few problems to get comfortable moving between the systems!

An owner tells you his dog weighs 64 lb. How many kg does it weigh?

$$64 \text{ lb} \times \frac{1 \text{ kg}}{2.2 \text{ lb}} = 29 \text{ kg}$$

Starting factor

Answer unit

Conversion factor

Here's another:

You are asked to give amoxicillin at a dose of 15 mg/kg to a cat that weighs 12 lb. How many mg of amoxicillin do you give?

$$12 \; \cancel{lb} \times \frac{1 \; \cancel{kg}}{2.2 \; \cancel{lb}} \times \frac{15 \; mg}{1 \; \cancel{kg}} = 82 \; mg$$

Starting factor

Answer unit

Conversion factors

As always, remember to arrange your conversion factors so that the desired units are left in the answer!

Let's do it again!

1. You ask a client to give her dog 90 mL of water every hour. How many ounces does this represent in the United States? In the United Kingdom?
2. You walk your dog 2 miles each day. How many km is this?
3. You are cutting disposable wrap for surgical packs and are asked to make them 1 yard long. How many cm is this?
4. A 2-lb ferret requires 10 mg/kg of a medication that comes in a strength of 1 mg/mL. How many mL should it receive?

ANSWERS

1. $90 \; \cancel{mL} \times \dfrac{1 \; oz}{30 \; \cancel{mL}} = 3 \; oz \; (US),$

   $90 \; \cancel{mL} \times \dfrac{1 \; oz}{28 \; \cancel{mL}} = 3.2 \; oz \; (UK)$

2. $2 \; \cancel{miles} \times \dfrac{1 \; km}{0.625 \; \cancel{miles}} = 3.2 \; km$

3. $1 \; \cancel{yard} \times \dfrac{91.44 \; cm}{1 \; \cancel{yard}} = 91.44 \; cm$

4. $2 \; \cancel{lb} \times \dfrac{1 \; \cancel{kg}}{2.2 \; \cancel{lb}} \times \dfrac{10 \; \cancel{mg}}{1 \; \cancel{kg}} \times \dfrac{1 \; mL}{1 \; \cancel{mg}} = 9.1 \; mL$

Multiple choice questions

1. An owner brings their puppy to you to be weighed. It weighs 7.4 kg. The owner wants to know the value in lb. What would be the weight in lb?

   a. 9.81 lb   b. 12.57 lb   c. 16.28 lb   d. 36.44 lb

2. A client runs 14.1 miles with her dog. What distance is the dog running in km?

   a. 7.5 km   b. 22.56 km   c. 26.8 km   d. 31.5 km

3. You need to administer medication to a rat weighing 1.75 kg. The dose for the medication is 7 mg/kg. How many mg do you administer?

   a. 8.5 mg   b. 10 mg   c. 11.5 mg   d. 12.25 mg

4. A dog weighs 2 stone, 4 lb. How much does it weigh in kg?

   a. 12.7 kg   b. 14.5 kg   c. 15.2 kg   d. 16.1 kg

5. A dog drinks 5 pints of water on a daily basis. How much is this in Imperial Litres to the nearest tenth?

   a. 2.9 L   b. 3.3 L   c. 3.5 L   d. 3.8 L

Answers

1. c. 16.28 lb
2. b. 22.56 km
3. d. 12.25 mg
4. b. 14.5 kg
5. a. 2.9 L

Chapter 5

Calculating medication dosages

Learning Objectives

- Types of oral medication
- Reading labels
- Calculating dosages of oral medications
- What is parenteral medication?
- Types of syringes
- Reconstituting powders
- Working with percent concentration
- Administration of insulin
- Calculating dosages of parenteral medication
- Clinical problems involving calculations

Types of oral medication

The majority of medications used in veterinary medicine are administered by the oral route (i.e. by mouth) and can come in various forms: tablets, capsules, liquid and powder. Tablets are manufactured with a specific amount of medication but can sometimes be divided into smaller portions if needed. Capsules do not lend themselves to dividing the dose, whereas liquids and powders can often be administered in various increments.

 The abbreviation for giving medication by mouth is p.o. (per os).

Some liquid medication is manufactured and stored in a powder form and then mixed with water or another solvent to make a liquid. In this case, the concentration of the medication can vary according to the amount of water or solvent added – be sure to follow directions carefully!

Oral medication labels

Reading labels carefully is extremely important in order to prevent dosing errors. The *three-way safety check* is a method of ensuring the correct medication is used each time. Remember to check the label for the correct drug and dosage when:

1. You *remove* it from the pharmacy shelf
2. You *dispense* the medication
3. You *replace* the medication.

Examine the label shown in Fig. 5.1 for important information to check each time you handle medication.

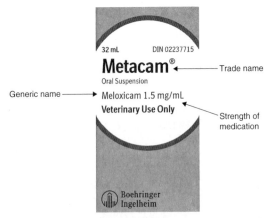

Fig. 5.1   Important information on the Metacam product packaging

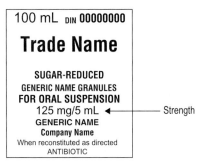

100 mL DIN **00000000**

Trade Name

SUGAR-REDUCED
GENERIC NAME GRANULES
FOR ORAL SUSPENSION
125 mg/5 mL ◄──────── Strength
GENERIC NAME
Company Name
When reconstituted as directed
ANTIBIOTIC

Fig. 5.2   Label information on powdered medication for reconstitution

Fig. 5.2 shows a label from a powdered antibiotic that must be reconstituted before use. With the medication in Fig. 5.2, once the label directions are followed, you will have 100 mL of medication, and each 5 mL will contain 125 mg. How much will each mL contain?

Using ratio and proportion: $\dfrac{5 \text{ mL}}{125 \text{ mg}} = \dfrac{1 \text{ mL}}{x \text{ mg}}$, $x = 25$ mg

Using dimensional analysis: $1 \text{ mL} \times \dfrac{125 \text{ mg}}{5 \text{ mL}} = 25$ mg

Let's use the two labels in Figs 5.1 and 5.2 to solve the following problems.

A 10-lb cat needs the antibiotic shown in Fig. 5.2 at 20 mg/kg twice daily. How many mL will you give at each dosing?

$$10 \text{ lb} \times \frac{1 \text{ kg}}{2.2 \text{ lb}} \times \frac{20 \text{ mg}}{1 \text{ kg}} \times \frac{5 \text{ mL}}{125 \text{ mg}} = 3.6 \text{ mL}$$

Notice how all the units except the desired answer units (mL) cancel out? The wonder of dimensional analysis!

Okay, we're on a roll, so let's do another….

A 65-lb Labrador retriever requires 0.1 mg/kg of meloxicam once daily. How many mL should it receive?

$$65 \text{ lb} \times \frac{1 \text{ kg}}{2.2 \text{ lb}} \times \frac{0.1 \text{ mg}}{1 \text{ kg}} \times \frac{1 \text{ mL}}{1.5 \text{ mg}} = 1.97 \text{ mL}$$

Of course, it is not practical to measure to one-hundredths of a mL, so you would give 2 mL. Note all the conversion factors that enable the desired answer units to appear in the answer.

 ## Let's do it again!

Use the two labels in Figs 5.1 and 5.2 to solve these clinical problems.

1. A 10-kg spaniel cross requires 22 mg/kg of antibiotic twice daily. How many mL are given at each treatment?
2. A 75-lb Doberman needs 0.15 mg/kg of meloxicam each morning. How many mL do you give?
3. A 6-lb cat is being treated for an abscess and needs 20 mg/kg of antibiotic twice daily for 5 days. How many mL will have to be dispensed?

ANSWERS

1. $10 \; \cancel{kg} \times \dfrac{22 \; \cancel{mg}}{1 \; \cancel{kg}} \times \dfrac{5 \; mL}{125 \; \cancel{mg}} = 8.8 \; mL$

2. $75 \; \cancel{lb} \times \dfrac{1 \; \cancel{kg}}{2.2 \; \cancel{lb}} \times \dfrac{0.15 \; \cancel{mg}}{1 \; \cancel{kg}} \times \dfrac{1 \; mL}{1.5 \; \cancel{mg}} = 3.4 \; mL$

3. $6 \; \cancel{lb} \times \dfrac{1 \; \cancel{kg}}{2.2 \; \cancel{lb}} \times \dfrac{20 \; \cancel{mg}}{1 \; \cancel{kg}} \times \dfrac{5 \; mL}{125 \; \cancel{mg}} \times \dfrac{2}{1 \; \cancel{day}} \times 5 \; \cancel{days} = 21.81 \, mL$

In this case, you would want to dispense at least 25 mL to ensure the client had enough medication to last.

What is parenteral administration?

The term *parenteral administration* refers to giving drugs 'in the space between the enteric canal and the surface of the body'. Essentially, this means injecting liquids with a needle into a vein (*intravenous*), into a muscle (*intramuscular*) or under the skin (*subcutaneous*). Rarely, drugs are injected into the peritoneal space – the space between the contents of the abdomen and the abdominal wall. There are advantages to parenteral administration, including almost 100% bioavailability of the drug, as it is not dependent on absorption through the intestine like an oral medication, and is not immediately affected by metabolism in the liver (remember anything absorbed from the intestine goes to the liver before ending up in the bloodstream). Disadvantages include potential pain for the patient and a higher degree of technical ability on the part of the clinical staff.

Abbreviations are:

Intravenous – i.v.
Intramuscular – i.m.
Subcutaneous – s.c. or s.q.
Intraperitoneal – i.p.

Types of syringe

The most commonly used syringe in small animal veterinary practice is the 3 mL (also known as the 3 cc) syringe (Fig. 5.3). This syringe is calibrated so that each increment equals 0.1 mL. Other sizes that are encountered are 5-, 6-, 10- and 12-mL syringes, in which each increment represents 0.2 mL. For smaller patients in which drug volumes are small, the tuberculin syringe is used: this is marked in 0.01-mL increments (Fig. 5.4). Occasionally, a 20-, 30- or 60-mL syringe is required. These are marked in 1-mL increments. When using a syringe, the volume is read at the top of the plunger.

Barking up the wrong tree

Be careful to use the correct syringe for the volume of medication you are administering. It is not accurate to measure 0.3 mL using a 12-mL syringe. A 3-mL or even a tuberculin syringe would be more appropriate.

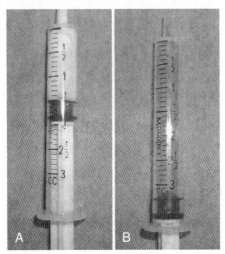

Fig. 5.3   The 3-mL syringe is calibrated in 0.1-mL increments and marked with numbers every 0.5 mL. A reading is taken at the level of the top of the plunger. **(A)** The syringe plunger has been withdrawn to 1.5 mL of medication

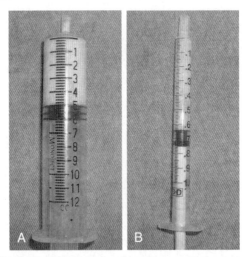

Fig. 5.4   **(A)** A 12-mL syringe showing plunger withdrawal to the 5-mL mark. **(B)** A tuberculin syringe showing plunger withdrawal to the 0.63-mL mark

Let's do it again!

What syringe size is appropriate for the following volumes?

1. 1.5 mL   2. 0.2 mL   3. 4.6 mL   4. 25 mL   5. 2.6 mL

ANSWERS

1. 3 mL   2. 1 mL (tuberculin)   3. 6 mL   4. 30 mL   5. 3 mL

Reconstituting powders

Some injectable drugs are stored as powders to increase their shelf life and reconstituted with sterile water or saline just before use. The label will contain directions for reconstituting that will give you the required concentration of drug. Cefazolin is an antibiotic that is often used prophylactically during orthopaedic procedures with instructions to give 20 mg/kg at induction of anaesthesia and then 20 mg/kg every 90 minutes until wound closure. The antibiotic comes as a dry powder in vials that contain 500, 1000 or 2000 mg of active drug. Also comes in 10g and 20g vials. Diluent (the saline or sterile water used to dissolve the antibiotic) is added in varying volumes, resulting in different concentrations (Table 5.1).

The powder takes up space so when diluent is added, the resultant volume is greater than just that of the diluent. In the first case above, the resultant concentration is 500 mg in 2.2 mL, which is 500 mg/2.2 mL = 225 mg/mL. In the second example, 1000 mg/3 mL = 333 mg/mL, and finally in the third example, 2000 mg/20.8 mL = 96 mg/mL.

Table 5.1 Reconstituting cefazolin at different concentrations

Vial size (mg)	Diluent added (mL)	Resultant volume (mL)	Concentration (mg/mL)
500	2	2.2	225
1000	2.5	3	333
2000	20	20.8	96

Let's do it again!

1. You have a 2-kg Chihuahua that requires surgery for a fractured leg. Using the 500-mg vial of cefazolin, how many mL of the antibiotic would you administer at induction?
2. A 55-kg yellow Labrador retriever requires shoulder surgery for osteochondrosis. How much of the reconstituted 1000-mg vial would you administer?

ANSWERS

1. $2 \text{ kg} \times \dfrac{20 \text{ mg}}{\text{kg}} \times \dfrac{1 \text{ mL}}{225 \text{ mg}} = 0.18 \text{ mL}$

2. $55 \text{ kg} \times \dfrac{20 \text{ mg}}{\text{kg}} \times \dfrac{1 \text{ mL}}{333 \text{ mg}} = 3.3 \text{ mL}$

Working with percent concentration

The concentrations of some injectable drugs are labelled in percent concentration rather than in mg/mL. One example is enrofloxacin, which comes in a liquid of 2.27%. This antibiotic is given by injection to start treatment (sometimes called a loading dose) at 2.5 mg/kg, and then oral tablets are used for the duration of the treatment. Remember that percent literally means 'per one hundred', so a concentration of 2.27% means that there are 2.27 parts of active drug for every 100 equivalent parts of solution. What is an 'equivalent part', you ask? One mL of water weighs 1 g and most medical solutions are nearly equivalent to water, so we assume they also have a mass of 1 g/mL.

For most solutions, remember:

$$1 \text{ mL} = 1 \text{ cc} = 1 \text{ g}$$

$$1\% = 1 \text{ g}/100 \text{ mL}$$

$$10\% = 10 \text{ g}/100 \text{ mL} \text{ (since 100 mL is the same as 100 g)}$$

In the example above, a 2.27% solution means there are 2.27 g of active ingredient in every 100 mL of solution. In other words:

$$\frac{2.27 \text{ g}}{100 \text{ mL}} \times \frac{1000 \text{ mg}}{1 \text{ g}} = 22.7 \text{ mg/mL}$$

If you have to give 2.5 mg/kg to a 32-kg dog, you would calculate it as follows:

$$\frac{2.5 \text{ mg}}{1 \text{ kg}} \times 32 \text{ kg} \times \frac{1 \text{ mL}}{22.7 \text{ mg}} = 3.5 \text{ mL}$$

 ## Barking up the wrong tree

There is a temptation to think of 1 mL of water as weighing 1 mg, as the words sound more similar than millilitre and gram. Don't get caught!

Administering insulin

Insulin is given to diabetic animals to replace the lack of natural insulin in their bodies. It is administered by clinical staff when a diabetic patient is in hospital but most often by the patient's owner at home. Insulin is measured in *international units* (IU) – a term that refers to a drug's *activity*, not its weight. Other drugs measured in this way include penicillin and heparin. Insulin comes in two common strengths: U-100, which has 100 units per mL, and U-40, which has 40 units per mL (Fig. 5.5).

Insulin must be administered with a specific type of syringe that is calibrated for the type of insulin used. U-100 syringes must *only* be used with U-100 insulin and U-40 syringes *only* with U-40

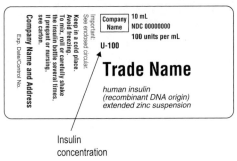

Insulin
concentration

Fig. 5.5 Humulin U-100 insulin labelling

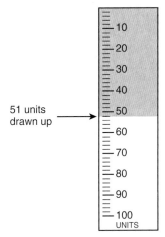

51 units
drawn up →

Fig. 5.6 A U-100 syringe barrel showing a reading of 51 units on the measurement scale. Standard insulin syringes are either in 1 mL, 0.5 mL or 0.3 mL sizes. Some are marked in 10 unit increments as shown, some are marked in 5 unit increments. Some also half half-unit marks, but the calibrations on both types are the same and always refer to the number of units drawn into the syringe

insulin (Fig. 5.6). Do not confuse insulin syringes with tuberculin syringes – they are not the same.

Insulin syringes are either 1 mL, 0.5 mL or 0.3 mL in size, but the calibrations always refer to the number of units drawn up into the syringe.

Barking up the wrong tree

What would happen if you used a U-100 syringe to draw up U-40 insulin? The U-40 insulin is $\dfrac{40 \text{ units/mL}}{100 \text{ units/mL}} = 40\%$ as strong as the U-100 insulin. Let's say you drew up 20 units of U-40 insulin with the U-100 syringe. You would actually have only 40% of 20 units, or 8 units.

Using a U-40 syringe for U-100 insulin would give you more insulin than you require, which could cause a severe reaction!

Let's try some clinical problems using insulin.

A 10-kg mixed-breed dog needs 4 IU/kg of insulin twice daily. How much insulin will the owner draw up each time?

$$10 \text{ kg} \times \frac{4 \text{ IU}}{1 \text{ kg}} = 40 \text{ IU}$$

A 60-lb German Shepherd requires 2 IU/kg of insulin twice daily. How much U-100 insulin will the owner need to use in 4 weeks?

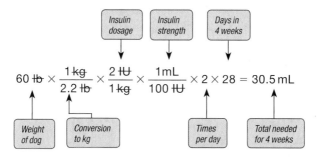

Notice once again that the conversion factor for the strength of the insulin is arranged so that the volume (mL) appears in the answer unit and all other units cancel.

Let's do it again!

1. A 12-lb cat needs 1 IU/kg of insulin once a day. Using U-40 insulin, how many units are given each day?
2. How many mL of U-100 insulin will be used in 1 week for a 35-lb Dachshund that is on a dose of 3 IU/kg twice daily?
3. If you accidentally used a U-40 syringe to draw up U-100 insulin, how many units would actually be contained in the syringe that is drawn to the 20-IU mark?

ANSWERS

1. $12 \; \cancel{lb} \times \dfrac{1 \; \cancel{kg}}{2.2 \; \cancel{lb}} \times \dfrac{1 \; IU}{\cancel{kg}} = 5.5 \; IU$

   Note that the type of insulin does not affect the number of units given, only the number of mL.

2. $35 \; \cancel{lb} \times \dfrac{1 \; \cancel{kg}}{2.2 \; \cancel{lb}} \times \dfrac{3 \; \cancel{IU}}{1 \; \cancel{kg}} \times \dfrac{1 \; mL}{100 \; \cancel{IU}} \times 2 \times 7 = 6.7 \; mL$

3. $\dfrac{100 \; units/mL}{40 \; units/mL} \times 20 \; IU = 50 \; IU$

Clinical problems using dosage calculations

Questions

1. 4 mg = how many g?
2. 5000 g = how many kg?
3. 120 mL = how many L?
4. 0.5 kg of water = how many mL?
5. A 20-lb dog needs 30 mg/kg of medication. How many mg of medication do you give?
6. A 40-kg dog needs 0.5 mg/kg of a medication that comes in 10-mg tablets. How many tablets will you give?

7. A 30-g mouse needs 400 µg/kg of a medication that comes in a liquid form with a strength of 0.1 mg/mL. How much will you give?

8. The dosage for a dog is 10 mg/kg. The dog weighs 25 kg and the medication comes in 100-mg tablets. How many tablets do you give?

9. Mrs. Smith's cat, weighing 5 kg needs insulin at 2 IU/kg. The insulin comes in a strength of 40 IU/mL. How much insulin do you give?

10. How many grams of dextrose does 350 mL of a 50% dextrose solution contain?

11. A 3.5-kg cat needs 20 mg/kg of liquid antibiotic that comes in a strength of 15 mg/mL. How many mL do you give (answer to nearest tenth)?

12. How many mg of acepromazine are in 1.2 mL of a 10 mg/mL solution?

13. A 13-kg dog needs 40 mg/kg of an antibiotic that comes in 250-mg capsules. How many capsules do you give?

14. If an injectable drug has a concentration of 10 mg/mL, how would you express this as a percentage concentration?

15. A 22-kg dog needs 2 mg/kg of a drug that comes as a 5% solution. How many mL do you give?

Answers

1. $4 \; \cancel{mg} \times \dfrac{1 \text{ g}}{1000 \; \cancel{mg}} = 0.004 \text{ g}$

2. $5000 \; \cancel{g} \times \dfrac{1 \text{ kg}}{1000 \; \cancel{g}} = 5 \text{ kg}$

3. $120 \; \cancel{mL} \times \dfrac{1 \text{ L}}{1000 \; \cancel{mL}} = 0.12 \text{ L}$

4. $0.5 \; \cancel{kg} \times \dfrac{1 \text{ mL}}{1 \; \cancel{g}} \times \dfrac{1000 \; \cancel{g}}{1 \; \cancel{kg}} = 500 \text{ mL}$

5. $20 \; \cancel{lb} \times \dfrac{1 \; \cancel{kg}}{2.2 \; \cancel{lb}} \times \dfrac{30 \text{ mg}}{1 \; \cancel{kg}} = 273 \text{ mg}$

6. $40 \text{ kg} \times \dfrac{0.5 \text{ mg}}{1 \text{ kg}} \times \dfrac{1 \text{ tab}}{10 \text{ mg}} = 2 \text{ tabs}$

7. $30 \text{ g} \times \dfrac{400 \text{ µg}}{1 \text{ kg}} \times \dfrac{1 \text{ kg}}{1000 \text{ g}} \times \dfrac{1 \text{ mL}}{0.1 \text{ mg}} \times \dfrac{1 \text{ mg}}{1000 \text{ µg}} = 0.12 \text{ mL}$

8. $25 \text{ kg} \times \dfrac{10 \text{ mg}}{1 \text{ kg}} \times \dfrac{1 \text{ tab}}{100 \text{ mg}} = 2.5 \text{ tabs}$

9. $5 \text{ kg} \times \dfrac{2 \text{ IU}}{1 \text{ kg}} \times \dfrac{1 \text{ mL}}{40 \text{ IU}} = 0.25 \text{ mL}$

10. $350 \text{ mL} \times \dfrac{50 \text{ g}}{100 \text{ mL}} = 175 \text{ g}, \quad \text{or} \dfrac{50 \text{ g}}{100 \text{ mL}} \times \dfrac{x \text{ g}}{350 \text{ mL}},$

    $x = 175 \text{ g}$

11. $3.5 \text{ kg} \times \dfrac{20 \text{ mg}}{1 \text{ kg}} \times \dfrac{1 \text{ mL}}{15 \text{ mg}} = 4.7 \text{ mL}$

12. $1.2 \text{ mL} \times \dfrac{10 \text{ mg}}{1 \text{ mL}} = 12 \text{ mg}, \quad \text{or} \dfrac{10 \text{ mg}}{1 \text{ mL}} = \dfrac{x \text{ mg}}{1.2 \text{ mL}}, \quad x = 12 \text{ mg}$

13. $13 \text{ kg} \times \dfrac{40 \text{ mg}}{1 \text{ kg}} \times \dfrac{1 \text{ capsule}}{250 \text{ mg}} =$

    2 capsules (you cannot split capsules)

14. (i) $\dfrac{10 \text{ mg}}{1 \text{ mL}} \times \dfrac{1 \text{ g}}{1000 \text{ mg}} = \dfrac{0.01 \text{ g}}{1 \text{ mL}}$

    (ii) $\dfrac{0.01 \text{ g}}{1 \text{ mL}} = \dfrac{x \text{ g}}{100 \text{ mL}}, \quad x = \dfrac{1 \text{ g}}{100 \text{ mL}} = 1\%$

15. $22 \text{ kg} \times \dfrac{2 \text{ mg}}{1 \text{ kg}} \times \dfrac{100 \text{ mL}}{5 \text{ g}} \times \dfrac{1 \text{ g}}{1000 \text{ mg}} = 0.88 \text{ mL}$

> 5% = 5 g/100 mL
> or 100 mL/5 g

Multiple choice questions

1. A 15.5-kg dog has been prescribed 20-mg tablets for 14 days. The dose is 2.5 mg/kg twice daily. What number of tablets are required?

   a. 14 tablets   b. 21 tablets   c. 28 tablets   d. 56 tablets

2. An owner calls in to collect a prescription of Cefazolin oral drops. The suspension, once reconstituted, contains 100 mg/mL. The dose rate for a 15-kg dog is 15 mg/kg twice daily. What is the daily amount the dog receives?

   a. 2.5 mL   b. 3.5 mL   c. 4.5 mL   d. 5.5 mL

3. Tablets are available in a strength of 4 mg and a cat weighing 8 kg requires a dose of 1 mg/kg three times daily for 10 days. How many tablets do you dispense to the cats owner?

   a. 6   b. 16   c. 20   d. 60

4. A 12-kg dog requires 25-mg tablets. The dosing instructions are 6 mg/kg daily (to the nearest whole tablet). How many tablets need to be dispensed for a 10-day course?

   a. 15   b. 20   c. 25   d. 30

5. Tablets come in a 30-mg strength and a 5-kg cat has received 20 tablets for a 10-day course. What is the dose rate?

   a. 5 mg/kg/day   b. 10 mg/kg/day
   c. 12 mg/kg/day   d. 15 mg/kg/day

Answers

1. d. 56 tablets
2. c. 4.5 mL
3. d. 60
4. d. 30
5. c. 12 mg/kg/day

Chapter 6

Solutions

Learning Objectives

● Making weaker solutions from stock solutions

Making weaker solutions from stock solutions

Many types of solutions that we use in the veterinary practice or research facility are concentrated to reduce the volume that needs to be shipped and stored. Before these *stock solutions* are used, they are diluted to the appropriate concentration. Many disinfectant solutions are diluted before use.

There is a simple concept that is helpful in determining how to dilute solutions:

$$C_1 \times V_1 = C_2 \times V_2$$

C_1 = concentration of solution 1; V_1 = volume of solution 1;

C_2 = concentration of solution 2; V_2 = volume of solution 2.

This equation simply tells us that, in terms of the active ingredient, a small volume of a concentrated solution is equal to a large volume of diluted solution. This is like money; a small number of large denominations is equal to an appropriate large number of small denominations. We also see this concept in laundry detergents where smaller volumes of concentrated detergents are often promoted over larger volumes of dilute solutions.

If we consider hydrogen peroxide, how much of a 10% concentration is equal to 1000 mL of a 1% concentration?

$C_1 = 1\%$; $V_1 = 1000$ mL; $C_2 = 10\%$; $V_2 =$ unknown

$$C_1V_1 = C_2V_2 \longrightarrow V_2 = \frac{C_1V_1}{C_2}$$

$$V_2 = \frac{(1\%)(1000 \text{ mL})}{10\%}, \quad V_2 = 100 \text{ mL}$$

Therefore 100 mL of a 10% concentration has the same amount of active ingredient as 1000 mL of a 1% solution.

We can use this relationship to determine how to dilute a stock solution. We need to know the starting and final concentration and how much of the dilute solution we are making.

How would you make 250 mL of a 2% hydrogen peroxide using a 10% stock solution?

$C_1 = 10\%$; $V_1 =$ unknown; $C_2 = 2\%$; $V_2 = 250$ mL

$$C_1V_1 = C_2V_2 \longrightarrow V_1 = \frac{C_2V_2}{C_1}$$

$$V_1 = \frac{(2\%)(250 \text{ mL})}{10\%}, \quad V_1 = 50 \text{ mL}$$

From our equation, we can see that 50 mL of a 10% solution will contain the same amount of active ingredient as 250 mL of a 2% solution. From this, we conclude that we need to take 50 mL of our 10% *stock solution* and dilute it up to 250 mL (i.e. add 200 mL of diluent) in order to make our *working solution*.

 ## Let's do it again!

1. From a 50% solution of dextrose, make 500 mL of a 5% solution.
2. Using a 70% solution of alcohol, make 200 mL of a 10% solution.

3. How much diluent do you add to make 100 mL of a 4% solution using a 20% stock solution?

ANSWERS

1. $C_1 = 50\%$; $V_1 =$ unknown; $C_2 = 5\%$; $V_2 = 500$ mL

$$C_1V_1 = C_2V_2 \longrightarrow V_1 = \frac{C_2 \times V_2}{C_1}$$

$$V_1 = \frac{(5\%) \times (500 \text{ mL})}{50\%}, \ V_1 = 50 \text{ mL}$$

Add 450 mL diluent to make 500 mL.

2. $C_1 = 70\%$; $V_1 =$ unknown; $C_2 = 10\%$; $V_2 = 200$ mL

$$V_1 = \frac{(10\%) \times (200 \text{ mL})}{70\%}, \ V_1 = 28.6 \text{ mL}$$

Add 171.4 mL of diluent.

3. $C_1 = 20\%$; $V_1 =$ unknown; $C_2 = 4\%$; $V_2 = 100$ mL

$$V_1 = \frac{(4\%) \times (100 \text{ mL})}{20\%}, \ V_1 = 20 \text{mL}$$

Add 80 mL of diluent.

We can use this concept for all dilutions of stock solutions, even if their concentrations are described in weight/volume units such as mg/mL.

Make 10 mL of a 10 mg/mL solution using a 100 mg/mL stock solution.

$$C_1 = 100 \text{ mg/mL}; V_1 = \text{unknown}; C_2 = 10 \text{ mg/mL}; V_2 = 10 \text{ mL}$$

$$C_1V_1 = C_2V_2 \longrightarrow V_1 = \frac{C_2V_2}{C_1}$$

$$V_1 = \frac{(10 \text{ mg/mL})(10 \text{ mL})}{100 \text{ mg/mL}}, \quad V_1 = 1 \text{ mL}$$

We take 1 mL of the 100 mg/mL stock solution and add 9 mL of diluent to make 10 mL of a 10 mg/mL solution.

Multiple choice questions

1. How many mg of active ingredient in 1 mL of a 0.9% solution?
   a. 0.09 mg   b. 0.9 mg   c. 9 mg   d. 90 mg

2. If 150 mL of a solution contains 15 g, how many mg will 6 mL contain?
   a. 0.6 mg   b. 6 mg   c. 60 mg   d. 600 mg

3. How much diluent is required to make 200 mL of a 2% solution from a stock solution of 20%?
   a. 180 mL   b. 18 mL   c. 1.8 mL   d. 0.18 mL

4. If you have a 16% solution, how many mg of active ingredient is contained in each mL?
   a. 0.16 mg   b. 1.6 mg   c. 16 mg   d. 160 mg

5. You require 20 mL of a 15% solution. You have a stock solution available to you in an 80% strength. How much of the 80% stock solution will you need?
   a. 3.75 mL   b. 13.75 mL   c. 23.75 mL   d. 33.75 mL

Answers

1. c. 9 mg
2. a. 0.6 mg
3. a. 180 mL
4. d. 160 mg
5. a. 3.75 mL

Chapter **7**

Intravenous fluids and constant rate infusions

Learning Objectives

- Understanding rates of fluid administration
- Determining how to calculate flow rates
- Using fluid administration sets
- Determining how to calculate drip rates
- Understand what is meant by constant rate infusion
- Determining rates of drug infusion
- Determining amount of drug to add to fluids

Intravenous fluid administration

Intravenous (i.v.) fluids are used to provide water, electrolytes, energy and, often, medication to patients. This is frequently necessary when oral administration is not appropriate or is insufficient to meet the patient's needs. One example would be a puppy suffering from parvovirus enteritis, which can cause severe vomiting and diarrhoea leading to dehydration. Attempting to give water and medicine orally is ineffective as it simply causes more vomiting and will not be absorbed.

There are many different types of i.v. fluids, but all are administered through a catheter (needle) placed in a vein. They must be administered at an appropriate rate to meet the patient's needs and yet not so quickly as to cause fluid overload which can cause congestion of the lungs and decrease ventilation.

Flow rates

A flow rate implies a volume of a substance delivered over a period of time. Rates are often expressed as a fraction in which the substance being delivered is the numerator of the fraction and time is the denominator. In veterinary medicine, the two most common flow rates are mL of i.v. fluids per hour (mL/h) and L of oxygen per minute (L/min) during anaesthesia. Rates can be described in more than one way to include different units of time and also to take into account the dosage required based on body weight. Intravenous fluid rates can be described as mL/h, mL/min or mL/24 h (i.e. volume delivered in 1 day). We can also describe i.v. fluid rates based on the weight of the patient – mL/kg/unit of time. An example would be an order to provide an i.v. fluid rate of 10 mL/kg/h during surgery. In other words, for every kg of body weight, 10 mL of fluid must be delivered every hour. In this rate, the denominator of the equation has a combined unit of kg/h.

Let's try some problems using i.v. flow rates.

A dehydrated puppy needs 10 mL/h. What volume of fluids will the puppy receive in 24 hours?

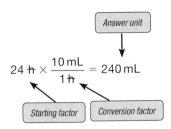

You will see that dimensional analysis works very well for flow rate problems, in this case turning our starting factor of 24 hours into our answer unit of 240 mL. Ratio and proportion can also be used:

$$\frac{10\ mL}{1\ h} = \frac{x\ mL}{24\ h}, \quad x = 240\ mL$$

Often it is necessary to calculate flow rates based on the *weight* of the patient.

If a 5-kg cat requires 2 mL/kg every hour, what is the flow rate per hour?

$$5\ \cancel{kg} \times \frac{2\ mL}{1\ \cancel{kg}\text{-h}} = \frac{10\ mL}{1\ h}$$

Note that the kg units cancel, leaving us with the desired answer units: mL/h.

Here's another example:

A 50-kg Doberman needs 50 mL/kg every 24 hours. What is the flow rate per hour?

$$50\ \cancel{kg} \times \frac{50\ mL}{\cancel{kg}\text{-}24\ h} = \frac{2500\ mL}{24\ h} = \frac{104\ mL}{1\ h}$$

If we wanted to determine the flow rate per minute, we simply add another conversion factor:

$$\frac{104\ mL}{1\ \cancel{h}} \times \frac{1\ \cancel{h}}{60\ min} = \frac{1.73\ mL}{1\ min}$$

 Let's do it again!

- 1. A 10-kg dog needs i.v. fluids of 10 mL/kg/h during surgery. What is the flow rate in mL/h? What is the rate in mL/min?
- 2. A 10-lb cat is on a flow rate of 20 mL/kg/h. How much will it receive in 3 hours?
- 3. A 20-kg dog needs fluids at a rate of 60 mL/kg/24 h. What is the flow rate in mL/h?

ANSWERS

1. $10 \; \cancel{kg} \times \dfrac{10 \; mL}{\cancel{kg}\text{-}h} = \dfrac{100 \; mL}{h}$, $10 \; \cancel{kg} \times \dfrac{10 \; mL}{\cancel{kg}\text{-}\cancel{h}} \times \dfrac{1 \; \cancel{h}}{60 \; min} = \dfrac{1.67 \; mL}{min}$

2. $10 \; \cancel{lb} \times \dfrac{1 \; \cancel{kg}}{2.2 \; \cancel{lb}} \times \dfrac{20 \; mL}{\cancel{kg}\text{-}\cancel{h}} \times 3 \; \cancel{h} = 272.7 \; mL$

3. $20 \; \cancel{kg} \times \dfrac{60 \; mL}{\cancel{kg}\text{-}24 \; h} = \dfrac{50 \; mL}{h}$

Fluid administration sets

Intravenous fluids are administered through plastic tubing with a *drip chamber* and a *roller clamp* (Fig. 7.1). The drip chamber is fed by a small metal tube that delivers a constant size of drop and prevents air from entering into the patient's bloodstream. Remember the i.v. route allows fluids and medication to be immediately available to the body. Intravenous fluids are used to support blood pressure, combat dehydration, restore electrolyte disturbances and to deliver medication. Intravenous sets used for small patients (under 7 kg) have a drip tube that provides 60 drops (abbreviated gtt which comes from the Latin word gutta which means drop) per mL (60 gtt/mL). Other sets for larger patients give 10 gtt/mL or 15 gtt/mL.

Adjusting the roller clamp will either increase or decrease the rate at which drops fall into the drip chamber and down the tube into the patient. We adjust this clamp until the desired number of drops per minute (gtt/min) is achieved. Typically, the number of drops in 15 seconds is counted and then multiplied by 4 to give the number of drops per minute. As an example, if you wanted to provide a patient with 40 gtt/min, you would adjust the clamp until 10 drops fell in 15 seconds.

Drip rates

If we know the type of administration set being used, we can determine drip rates based on flow rates expressed in mL/h or mL/min. Here's an example:

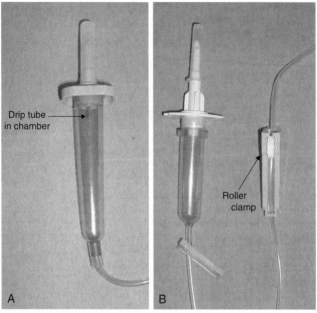

Drip tube in chamber

Roller clamp

A

B

Fig. 7.1 Fluid administration sets. **A**, A 60 gtt/mL set containing a small drip tube within the fluid chamber or reservoir. **B**, A 10 gtt/mL set showing the roller clamp that adjusts the drip rate

A dehydrated Persian cat requires fluids delivered at a rate of 20 mL/h. Using a 60 gtt/mL administration set, how will you set the drip rate in gtt/min?

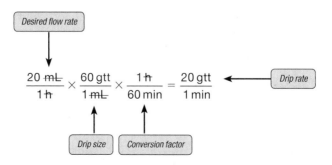

Desired flow rate

$$\frac{20 \text{ mL}}{1 \text{ h}} \times \frac{60 \text{ gtt}}{1 \text{ mL}} \times \frac{1 \text{ h}}{60 \text{ min}} = \frac{20 \text{ gtt}}{1 \text{ min}}$$

Drip rate

Drip size   Conversion factor

Our starting factor was the established flow rate and our answer units were gtt/min. The conversion factors included the drip chamber size and a time unit conversion.

Once again, we could use ratio and proportion but it would require more steps:

$$\frac{60 \text{ gtt}}{1 \text{ mL}} = \frac{x \text{ gtt}}{20 \text{ mL}}, \quad x = 1200 \text{ gtt in 20 mL}$$

$$\frac{1200 \text{ gtt}}{60 \text{ min}} = \frac{x \text{ gtt}}{1 \text{ min}}, \quad x = 20 \text{ gtt in 1 min}$$

Let's do a few more problems adding some other factors.

A 10-kg dog needs 10 mL/kg every hour during surgery. Using a 10 gtt/mL i.v. set, how will you set the rate in gtt/min?

$$10 \text{ kg} \times \frac{10 \text{ mL}}{\text{kg-h}} \times \frac{10 \text{ gtt}}{1 \text{ mL}} \times \frac{1 \text{ h}}{60 \text{ min}} = \frac{16.7 \text{ gtt}}{1 \text{ min}}$$

Of course, it is impossible to count 0.7 of a drop, so we always round up or down the number of drops. In this case we would set the drip rate at 17 gtt/min.

A 4-kg cat requires 50 mL/kg every 24 hours to maintain its hydration. Using a 60 gtt/mL i.v. set, how will you set the rate in gtt/min?

$$4 \text{ kg} \times \frac{50 \text{ mL}}{\text{kg-24 h}} \times \frac{60 \text{ gtt}}{1 \text{ mL}} \times \frac{1 \text{ h}}{60 \text{ min}} = \frac{8.3 \text{ gtt}}{1 \text{ min}} = 8 \text{ gtt/min}$$

↑

This conversion factor is the prescribed rate – for every 24 hours, give 50 mL per kg

Let's do it again!

- 1. A patient is to receive fluids of 40 mL/h. Using a 60 gtt/mL set, how will you set the rate in gtt/min?
- 2. A 45-kg dog requires maintenance fluids at 50 mL/kg every 24 hours. Using a 10 gtt/mL set, how will you set the rate in gtt/min?
- 3. You are asked to give fluids of 120 mL/kg/24 h to a 3.5-kg cat. How will you set the rate in gtt/min using a 60 gtt/mL set?

ANSWERS

1. $$\frac{40 \ \text{mL}}{\text{h}} \times \frac{60 \ \text{gtt}}{\text{mL}} \times \frac{1 \ \text{h}}{60 \ \text{min}} = \frac{40 \ \text{gtt}}{\text{min}}$$

2. $45 \ \text{kg} \times \dfrac{50 \ \text{mL}}{\text{kg-24 h}} \times \dfrac{10 \ \text{gtt}}{\text{mL}} \times \dfrac{1 \ \text{h}}{60 \ \text{min}} = \dfrac{15.6 \ \text{gtt}}{\text{min}}$; set it at

   16 gtt/min

3. $3.5 \ \text{kg} \times \dfrac{120 \ \text{mL}}{\text{kg-24 h}} \times \dfrac{60 \ \text{gtt}}{\text{mL}} \times \dfrac{1 \ \text{h}}{60 \ \text{min}} = \dfrac{17.5 \ \text{gtt}}{\text{min}}$; set it at

   18 gtt/min

Constant rate infusions

In most cases, medications are administered at set intervals throughout the day. For example, a dog may receive an antibiotic injection every 8 hours. The level of medication in the patient will rise to a peak and then start to fall as the body metabolizes and excretes it. Many medications have to reach a certain concentration in the bloodstream in order to be effective, so this waning of the concentration renders the medication ineffective. The faster the metabolism and excretion occurs, the more often the medication must be given in order to ensure therapeutic levels throughout the day. If the medication is given intravenously at a constant rate, the levels in the body stay the same at all times. This is important for some drugs used in intensive care situations and during anaesthesia. Examples of such drugs include metoclopramide, used to control vomiting, and lidocaine, used to control an irregular heartbeat. The dosage for these drugs is described as an amount delivered per kilogram of body weight per unit of time. For instance, the prescribed rate of metoclopramide infusion is 1–2 mg/kg/24 h.

Determining infusion rates

Using the prescribed dosage, we can calculate how much drug to infuse over a period of time. We start by determining the weight of the drug and then, taking into account the concentration of the drug, we calculate the volume of drug to use.

If a 10-kg dog requires 2 mg/kg of metoclopramide every 24 hours, how much drug do you infuse in 24 hours?

$$10 \; \cancel{kg} \times \frac{2 \; mg}{\cancel{kg}\text{-}24 \; h} = \frac{20 \; mg}{24 \; h}$$

If the concentration of the drug is 5 mg/mL, what volume is infused over 24 hours?

$$20 \; \cancel{mg} \times \frac{1 \; mL}{5 \; \cancel{mg}} = 4 \; mL$$

We could put all this information in one equation if the two questions were combined:

$$10 \; \cancel{kg} \times \frac{2 \; \cancel{mg}}{\cancel{kg}\text{-}24 \; h} \times \frac{1 \; mL}{5 \; \cancel{mg}} = \frac{4 \; mL}{24 \; h}$$

Let's do it again!

- 1. A 20-kg dog is prescribed a drug to be given at a constant rate infusion of 5 mg/kg every 24 hours. The drug has a strength of 10 mg/mL. What volume of drug is infused over 24 hours?
- 2. A drug with a concentration of 1 mg/mL was infused into a patient. The 4-kg patient received 15 mL of this drug in 10 hours. What was the infusion rate in mg/kg/h? Note: This is a similar question to the previous ones but 'in reverse'. Work backwards to find your answer.
- 3. A 24-lb dog needs a drug infused at a rate of 0.2 mg/kg/h. Using a drug with a strength of 5 mg/mL, how many mL of the drug will be needed for 12 hours?

ANSWERS

1. $20 \ \cancel{kg} \times \dfrac{5 \ \cancel{mg}}{\cancel{kg}\text{-}24 \ h} \times \dfrac{1 \ mL}{10 \ \cancel{mg}} = \dfrac{10 \ mL}{24 \ h}$

2. $\dfrac{15 \ \cancel{mL}}{4 \ kg\text{-}10 \ h} \times \dfrac{1 \ mg}{\cancel{mL}} = \dfrac{0.38 \ mg}{kg\text{-}h}$

3. $24 \ \cancel{lb} \times \dfrac{1 \ kg}{2.2 \ \cancel{lb}} \times \dfrac{0.2 \ \cancel{mg}}{\cancel{kg}\text{-}\cancel{h}} \times \dfrac{1 \ mL}{5 \ \cancel{mg}} \times 12 \ \cancel{h} = 5.2 \ mL$

Adding drugs to i.v. fluids

The volume of undiluted drug administered by constant rate infusion is usually very small. In order to accurately deliver the drug over a period of time, it has to be diluted with i.v. fluids. Most patients that require constant rate infusions are placed on i.v. fluids anyway due to the serious nature of their disease. The trick is to match the amount of drug with the rate of fluid administration and then determine the volume of drug to add to a set amount of fluids.

Example

In the example above, we decided that the amount of drug that needs to be delivered in a set period of time is 10 mL. During this same period of time, assume 1000 mL of fluids must be administered (based on the patient's fluid losses and maintenance requirements). We must therefore add 10 mL of the drug to 1000 mL of fluids and administer that over the time period in order to meet our objectives.

 To be totally accurate, we would add the 10 mL of the drug to 990 mL of fluids – to obtain 1000 mL of total fluids administered. When a small volume of drug is added to a large volume of fluid, however, this is not necessary, but it should be taken into account with larger volumes of drugs or small volumes of fluids.

A 4-kg cat is prescribed a drug at 2 mg/kg/24 h and the drug has a concentration of 1 mg/mL. The drug is to be added to a 500 mL bag of saline solution that is given at a rate to meet maintenance requirements of 60 mL/kg/24 h. How much of the drug is added to the 500 mL bag of fluids and at what rate is the fluid/drug mixture given?

Volume of drug to be administered over 24 hours:

$$4 \; \cancel{kg} \; \frac{2 \; \cancel{mg}}{\cancel{kg}\text{-}24 \; h} \times \frac{1 \; mL}{1 \; \cancel{mg}} = \frac{8 \; mL}{24 \; h}$$

Volume of fluids to be administered over 24 hours:

$$4 \; \cancel{kg} \; \frac{60 \; mL}{\cancel{kg}\text{-}24 \; h} = \frac{240 \; mL}{24 \; h}$$

We see that, in a 24 hour period, 8 mL of the drug and 240 mL of fluids will be administered. We can determine the amount to add to 500 mL of fluid using this relationship:

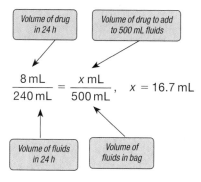

We would add 16.7 mL of the drug to 483.3 mL (500 − 16.7) of i.v. fluids and then administer the combination at the rate prescribed:

$$\frac{240\ mL}{24\ h} = \frac{10\ mL}{h}$$

If we do not have an infusion pump available and are using a 60 gtt/mL i.v. set, the drip rate would be:

$$\frac{10\ \cancel{mL}}{1\ \cancel{h}} \times \frac{60\ gtt}{1\ \cancel{mL}} \times \frac{1\ \cancel{h}}{60\ min} = \frac{10\ gtt}{min}$$

We can check our answer by working backwards:

In 240 mL of fluid (the amount administered in 24 hours), we have 8 mL of drug. The concentration of the drug is 1 mg/mL, so we have 8 mg of the drug given in 24 hours.

The weight of the patient is 4 kg, so we are giving 2 mg/kg every 24 hours.

 These problems can be quite complex, so it is worth checking your answer in this fashion before adding the drug.

Let's do it again!

1. A 10-kg dog requires a drug to be given by continuous infusion at a rate of 1 mg/kg/h using a maintenance fluid rate of 50 mL/kg over 24 hours. How many mg of drug are to be added to 1 L of fluids?

2. A 10-kg dog is receiving fluids at a rate of 40 mL/h. It needs a drug added to 500 mL of fluids so that it receives 2 mg/kg each hour. The drug has a strength of 2%. What volume of drug will you add?

3. A 5-kg diabetic cat needs a constant infusion of insulin of 0.1 units/kg each hour. It is on maintenance fluids of 60 mL/kg every 24 hours and a 60 gtt/mL drip set is in use. The insulin concentration is 40 IU/mL. How many mL of insulin will you add to a 250 mL bag of fluids?

ANSWERS

1. Amount of drug needed in 24 hours:

$$10 \; \cancel{kg} \times \frac{1\,mg}{\cancel{kg}\text{-}\cancel{h}} \times 24 \; \cancel{h} = 240 \; mg$$

Volume of fluid needed in 24 hours:

$$10 \; \cancel{kg} \times \frac{50 \; mL}{\cancel{kg}\text{-}24\,h} = \frac{500 \; mL}{24 \; h}$$

In 500 mL of fluid, you would need 240 mg of drug; therefore, in 1 L (1000 mL), you would need 480 mg of drug.

2. Volume of drug needed in 1 hour:

$$10 \; \cancel{kg} \times \frac{2 \; \cancel{mg}}{\cancel{kg}\text{-}h} \times \frac{100 \; mL}{2 \; \cancel{g}} \times \frac{1\,\cancel{g}}{1000 \; \cancel{mg}} = \frac{1 \; mL}{h}$$

$$\boxed{2\% = 2\,g \text{ for every } 100\,mL}$$

Volume of fluid to be given in 1 hour: 40 mL
Volume of drug added to 500 mL:

$$\frac{1\ mL}{40\ mL} = \frac{x\ mL}{500\ mL},\ x = 12.5\ mL$$

Add 12.5 mL of drug to 487.5 mL of fluid and infuse at a rate of 40 mL/h.

3. Volume of insulin needed in 24 hours:

$$5\ \cancel{kg} \times \frac{0.1\ \cancel{units}}{\cancel{kg}\text{-}\cancel{h}} \times 24\ \cancel{h} \times \frac{1\ mL}{40\ \cancel{units}} = 0.3\ mL$$

Volume of fluid needed in 24 hours:

$$5\ \cancel{kg} \times \frac{60\ mL}{\cancel{kg}\text{-}24\ h} = \frac{300\ mL}{24\ h}$$

Volume of insulin per 250 mL:

$$\frac{0.3\ mL}{300\ mL} = \frac{x\ mL}{250\ mL},\ x = 0.25\ mL$$

Multiple choice questions

1. Your 23-kg patient has been receiving fluid at a rate of 60 mL/kg/24 h for the last 10 hours. How much fluid has he received?
   a. 335 mL   b. 435 mL   c. 575 mL   d. 625 mL

2. A 9-kg dog requires 40 mL/kg of fluid every 24 hours. How much fluid will it have received after 13 hours?
   a. 25 mL   b. 60 mL   c. 195 mL   d. 360 mL

3. A 14-kg dog is receiving 50 mL/kg/24 h of i.v. fluids. How many mL does it receive per minute?
   a. 0.5 mL   b. 5 mL   c. 15 mL   d. 29 mL

4. A 25-kg dog is receiving fluid at 6 mL/kg/h. How many mL will the dog have received after 45 minutes?
   a. 112.5 mL   b. 222.5 mL   c. 352.5 mL   d. 422.5 mL

5. How much fluid would a 21-kg dog receive in 8 hours if the fluid was given at a rate of 40 mL/kg/24 h?

a. 280 mL   b. 270 mL   c. 260 mL   d. 250 mL

Answers

1. c. 575 mL
2. c. 195 mL
3. a. 0.5 mL
4. a. 112.5 mL
5. a. 280 mL

Chapter **8**

Dilutions

Learning Objectives

- What is a dilution?
- Determining the final concentration in a dilution
- Dilution series
- Serial dilutions
- Immunology applications
- Microbiology applications
- Haematology applications

What is a dilution?

A dilution refers to a *weakened solution*. We have seen that some solutions used in veterinary practice come in a concentrated form (stock solution) and must be diluted before use (working solution).

Other examples of using dilutions include performing a complete blood count (CBC) which is a measure of the number of different types of red and white blood cells in circulation. Due to such large numbers of these cells in the blood, we cannot count them on a microscope slide therefore, we dilute the blood sample first, then cells are counted and the actual number of cells in the undiluted sample is calculated by *extrapolation*.

Microbiology applications include diluting a sample and counting the number of bacterial colonies formed and extrapolating back to the original sample. In immunology, the number of antibodies in serum is determined by a series of diluted serum samples. In order to perform these calculations, we need to understand the relationship between a diluted sample and the original sample.

 The preferred method of describing a dilution is: the number of parts of the substance being diluted in the total number of parts in the final product.

For instance, if I take 1 part serum and dilute it so that the total number of parts is 10, I have made a one-in-ten dilution. I may do this by taking 1 mL of serum and adding 9 mL of saline or I may take 10 mL of serum and add 90 mL of saline. In the first instance, I would have 10 mL of a one-in-ten dilution of serum, and in the second I would have 100 mL.

Dilutions are written as fractions with the substance being diluted as the numerator and the total volume of the solution as the denominator:

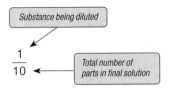

Substance being diluted

$$\frac{1}{10}$$

Total number of parts in final solution

In this example, the dilution is $\frac{1}{10}$ or, remembering the principles we learned in Chapter 1, we could also express this as 0.1 or 10^{-1}.

Generally, the dilution is expressed so that the numerator is one. If we took 5 parts of serum and diluted it with 5 parts of saline, the dilution would be $\frac{5}{10}$, but we would express this as $\frac{1}{2}$.

Barking up the wrong tree

You may see dilutions expressed as a ratio. For instance, in the $\frac{1}{10}$ serum *in* saline example above, there is 1 part serum to 9 parts saline, or a 1:9 serum *to* saline ratio. Be careful not to confuse these two descriptions of the same solution.

Determining dilution concentrations

If we know the original concentration of a solution and how the solution is diluted, we can determine the final concentration of the diluted solution:

Original concentration × *Dilution* = *Final concentration*

$OC \times D = FC$

If we use the $\frac{1}{10}$ serum sample, the original concentration is 100%, the dilution is $\frac{1}{10}$ and so the final concentration is:

$$100\% \times \frac{1}{10} = 10\%$$

Let's do it again!

1. A 10% saline solution is diluted $\frac{1}{10}$. What is the final concentration?
2. A solution that was diluted $\frac{1}{5}$ has a concentration of 10%. What was the original concentration?

3. If a drug with a concentration of 100 mg/mL is diluted $\frac{1}{20}$, what is the final concentration?

4. A stock solution with a concentration of 70% is diluted and the working solution has a concentration of 3.5%. How was it diluted?

ANSWERS

1. $OC \times D = FC$, $10\% \times \frac{1}{10} = 1\%$

2. $OC \times D = FC$, $OC = \frac{FC}{D}$, $OC = 10\% \div \frac{1}{5}$, $OC = 10\% \times \frac{5}{1} = 50\%$

3. $OC \times D = FC$, $100 \text{ mg/mL} \times \frac{1}{20} = 5 \text{ mg/mL}$

4. $OC \times D = FC$, $D = \frac{FC}{OC}$, $D = \frac{3.5\%}{70\%} = \frac{1}{20} = 0.05 = 5 \times 10^{-2}$

   (All are expressions of the same number.)

Dilution series

In some applications, we would like to make a series of dilutions rather than just a single dilution. There are two ways to do this. We can go to the original solution each time – *independent dilutions* – or we can use the first dilution to make a second dilution – *dependent dilutions* (a dilution of a dilution).

Independent dilutions

Let's say we have a serum sample and we want to make a $\frac{1}{5}$, $\frac{1}{10}$ and $\frac{1}{100}$ dilution. To accomplish this with independent dilutions, we would:

1. Take 1 part serum and dilute up to 5 parts with saline = $\frac{1}{5}$
2. Take 1 part serum and dilute up to 10 parts with saline = $\frac{1}{10}$
3. Take 1 part serum and dilute up to 100 parts with saline = $\frac{1}{100}$

Dependent dilutions

If we want to make the same dilutions but only want to use the serum once, we can make dependent dilutions:

1. Take 1 part serum and dilute up to 5 parts with saline = $\frac{1}{5}$
2. Take 1 part of the $\frac{1}{5}$ dilution and dilute up to 2 parts with saline:
   $$\frac{1}{5} \times \frac{1}{2} = \frac{1}{10}$$
3. Take 1 part of the $\frac{1}{10}$ dilution and dilute up to 10 parts with saline:
   $$\frac{1}{10} \times \frac{1}{10} = \frac{1}{100}$$

 You can see that in a dependent dilution the final dilution is the product of the series of dilutions:

Final dilution = dilution 1 × dilution 2 × dilution 3 × ...

 # Let's do it again!

1. A solution was diluted $\frac{1}{2}$, then again $\frac{1}{4}$, then again $\frac{1}{10}$. What is in the final dilution?
2. A solution was diluted once and then rediluted $\frac{1}{10}$ and again $\frac{1}{5}$. If the final solution was a $\frac{1}{100}$ dilution, how was the first solution diluted?
3. A drug with a concentration of 1000 mg/mL was diluted $\frac{1}{10}$, then rediluted $\frac{1}{5}$. What is the final concentration?

ANSWERS

1. $\dfrac{1}{2} \times \dfrac{1}{4} \times \dfrac{1}{10} = \dfrac{1}{80}$

2. *Final dilution = dilution 1 × dilution 2 × dilution 3*
   Dilution 1 = final dilution ÷ (dilution 2 × dilution 3)

   $Dilution\ 1 = \dfrac{1}{100} \div \left(\dfrac{1}{10} \times \dfrac{1}{5} \right) = \dfrac{1}{120} \div \dfrac{1}{50} = \dfrac{1}{100} \times \dfrac{50}{1} = \dfrac{1}{2}$

3. $OC \times D = FC$, 1000 mg/mL $\times \left(\dfrac{1}{10} \times \dfrac{1}{5} \right) = 20$ mg/mL

Serial dilutions

Many laboratory procedures involve a series of dependent dilutions in which each dilution is of the same magnitude. This is known as a serial dilution. For instance, if a serum sample is diluted $\frac{1}{10}$, rediluted $\frac{1}{10}$, then rediluted again $\frac{1}{10}$, we would call this a serial dilution. The term *fold* is often used to describe a serial dilution. In this example, we have a 10-fold dilution of serum. Sometimes, the first dilution is different than the rest, so if the first dilution in our example had been $\frac{1}{2}$, we would call it a 10-fold dilution that started at 2.

Once again, by knowing the original concentration and the dilutions, we can determine the concentration of the sample at any step along the way (Fig. 8.1).

Let's say we had a drug that came in a very concentrated form that was used for horses and we wanted to make a diluted form for use in birds. We could use a serial dilution to accomplish this.

How would you make a serial dilution for ivermectin 10 mg/mL so that the final concentration was 0.1 mg/mL?

From our equation: $OC \times dilution = FC$, we determine that the dilution has to be:

$$Dilution = \frac{FC}{OC} = \frac{0.1\,mg/mL}{10\,mg/mL} = \frac{1}{100}$$

	Serum	$\frac{1}{10}$ dilution	$\frac{1}{10}$ dilution	$\frac{1}{10}$ dilution
Total dilution	None	$\frac{1}{10}$	$\frac{1}{100}$	$\frac{1}{1000}$
Concentration	100%	10%	1%	0.1%

Fig. 8.1 Successive dilutions of $\frac{1}{10}$

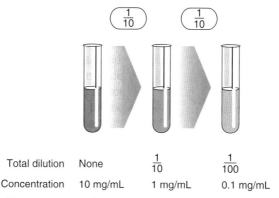

Total dilution	None	$\frac{1}{10}$	$\frac{1}{100}$
Concentration	10 mg/mL	1 mg/mL	0.1 mg/mL

Fig. 8.2 Two successive $\frac{1}{10}$ dilution steps

This can be accomplished in two steps using a $\frac{1}{10}$ serial dilution (Fig. 8.2).

It is possible to perform this dilution in just one step (a $\frac{1}{100}$ dilution), but it is difficult to be accurate when measuring small amounts. If we were only making 10 mL of the final drug, we would have to measure 0.1 mL to do it in one step, whereas if we do it in two steps, our smallest measure would be 1 mL which is much less prone to error.

Immunology applications

A *titre* is the term used for measuring the number of antibodies in a serum sample and is used to determine if a patient has been exposed to a particular microorganism or a vaccine. A titre is determined by setting up a serial dilution of a serum sample and then placing into each sample a known amount of antigen tied to a molecule that causes a reaction in the solution. The titre is the greatest dilution producing a positive reaction. You can see that if a patient has a great immune response to a microorganism or a vaccine, the positive reaction will be seen in a very dilute sample of serum.

Say a two-fold serial dilution of serum is set up and a positive reaction is observed in the $\frac{1}{2}$ and $\frac{1}{4}$ dilutions but not in the other dilutions. The titre is $\frac{1}{4}$ – the greatest dilution producing a positive reaction. Sometimes a titre is reported as the reciprocal of the dilution – in this case 4. A high titre (a very dilute sample) indicates a strong response by the immune system.

Let's do it again!

1. Starting with a tube of a 50% solution, what is the concentration in tube number 5 if the solution undergoes a 10-fold serial dilution?

2. A four-fold dilution is carried out on a drug. The concentration after four steps is 0.05 mg/mL. What was the original concentration?

3. A five-fold serial dilution of serum is set up and the last positive reaction to an antigen is found in the fourth tube. What is the titre? (Count the first tube as the first dilution.)

ANSWERS

1. *OC × dilution (dilution 1 × dilution 2 ...) = FC*

   $50\% \times \left(\frac{1}{10} \times \frac{1}{10} \times \frac{1}{10} \times \frac{1}{10} \right) = 50\% \times \frac{1}{10,000} = 50\% \times 10^{-4}$

   $= 5 \times 10^{-3}\% = 0.005\%$

2. *OC × D = FC; OC* $= \dfrac{FC}{D} = \dfrac{0.05 \text{ mg/mL}}{\left(\frac{1}{4} \times \frac{1}{4} \times \frac{1}{4} \times \frac{1}{4} \right)} = \dfrac{0.05 \text{ mg/mL}}{\left(\frac{1}{256} \right)}$

   $= 0.05 \text{ mg/mL} \times 256 = 12.8 \text{ mg/mL}$

3. *Total dilution = dilution 1 × dilution 2 × dilution 3 × dilution 4*

   $= \frac{1}{5} \times \frac{1}{5} \times \frac{1}{5} \times \frac{1}{5} = \frac{1}{625}$

   The titre is 1/625 (or, as often expressed, 625).

Microbiology applications

One method to determine how susceptible a microorganism is to an antibiotic is called the broth dilution susceptibility test. This involves a series of test tubes with dilutions of an antibiotic. A standardized amount of an organism is inoculated into the tubes. The first tube in which there is no growth of the organism, evidenced by a clear solution, is the minimum inhibitory concentration (MIC); in other words, the most dilute amount of antibiotic that is capable of preventing growth of the organism. This determines the type and dosage of antibiotic that needs to be given for a particular infectious organism.

Note the similarity to the titre test in immunology. Here the positive reaction is indicated by no growth of the organism and thus a clear solution (Fig. 8.3).

A solution of 20 mg/mL of an antibiotic is diluted $\frac{1}{2}$, then rediluted $\frac{1}{2}$. This is the last clear solution of the antibiotic. What is the MIC?

$$(OC = 20 \text{ mg/mL}) \times \left(Dilution = \frac{1}{2} \times \frac{1}{2} = \frac{1}{4} \right) = (FC = 5 \text{ mg/mL})$$

The MIC is 5 mg/mL.

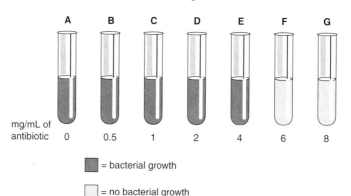

	A	B	C	D	E	F	G
mg/mL of antibiotic	0	0.5	1	2	4	6	8

■ = bacterial growth

☐ = no bacterial growth

Fig. 8.3 A broth dilution susceptibility test. Tube G has an antibiotic concentration of 8 mg/mL. A series of dilutions of antibiotic is performed and then a standard amount of organism is inoculated into each of tubes A–G. Tube F, with 6 mg/mL antibiotic, demonstrates the minimum inhibitory concentration (MIC) of antibiotic for this organism since the next dilution below it allows bacterial growth to occur.

Another application in microbiology is performing colony counts on a microorganism broth culture. A very small volume of the broth culture is plated on to a culture medium using a *loop* that holds a standard volume. After 24–48 hours, the number of *colony forming units (cfu)* is counted. Each colony represents one original bacterium.

It is often necessary to dilute the broth culture before plating it out otherwise too many colonies will form, making counting difficult. We take this dilution, along with the volume of the diluted broth culture that is plated, into account when determining the number of colony forming units per litre (cfu/L).

A bacterial culture is diluted $\frac{1}{1000}$ (10^{-3}) and then 0.05 mL of this diluted sample is plated onto a culture plate. After 48 hours, 75 cfu are counted. What was the concentration of organisms (cfu/L) in the original culture?

Original concentration × dilution = final concentration

We are looking for the original concentration, so we can rearrange the above equation:

$$Original\ concentration = \frac{final\ concentration}{dilution}$$

$$Final\ concentration = \frac{75\ cfu}{0.05\ mL}, \quad Dilution = \frac{1}{1000}$$

$$Original\ concentration = \frac{\left(\dfrac{75\ cfu}{0.05\ mL}\right)}{\left(\dfrac{1}{1000}\right)}$$

 Remember: when dividing by a fraction, simply multiply by the reciprocal. In this case, dividing by $\frac{1}{1000}$ is the same as multiplying by 1000.

$$Original\ concentration = \frac{75\ cfu}{0.05\ mL} \times \frac{1000}{1} = \frac{75,000\ cfu}{0.05\ mL}$$

$$= \frac{1,500,000\ cfu}{1\ mL}$$

This gives us the number of cfu per mL, but we need to report it in cfu per L, so let's use some dimensional analysis:

$$\frac{1,500,000 \text{ cfu}}{1 \text{ mL}} \times \frac{1000 \text{ mL}}{1 \text{ L}} = \frac{1,500,000,000 \text{ cfu}}{1 \text{ L}}$$

Such a large number is best expressed in scientific notation: 1.5×10^9 cfu/L.

Haematology applications

As a veterinary technician or nurse, one of the most commonly encountered diagnostic tests is the CBC. This involves taking a sample of blood and estimating the number of red blood cells, white blood cells and each type of white blood cell. The concentration of cells in the blood is very high, so we need to dilute the blood sample in order to count a smaller number and then extrapolate back to the original sample.

Dilution is carried out by drawing a set quantity of blood into a pipette and adding a known amount of diluent. There are several types of diluting pipettes but the most common one creates a $\frac{1}{100}$ dilution. Once the blood is diluted, a standard volume of the diluted sample is examined under the microscope and the number of cells counted. The result is a number of cells in a volume of sample – a concentration.

Haemocytometers

How do we ensure a standard volume is used each time? A special microscope slide called a haemocytometer is used, the most common of which is called the *Neubauer haemocytometer*. This slide has an area marked with various sizes of squares (Fig. 8.4) and it is also 0.1 mm in depth. This allows a set volume (area × depth) to be scanned and the number of cells counted.

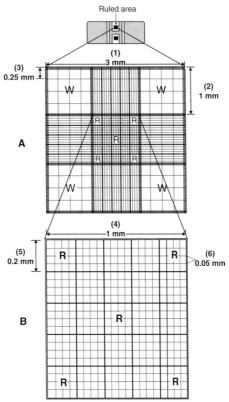

Fig. 8.4   The Neubauer haemocytometer counting area is divided into nine large squares, each measuring 1 mm × 1 mm (or 1 mm²). These larger squares are designated 'W' and are used to count white blood cells. If four of these squares are used, and the number of white cells in them counted, then the volume used is: 4 × 1 mm² × 0.1 mm (depth) = 0.4 mm³.

The central square is divided into 25 smaller squares, designated 'R', which are used to count red blood cells. Each R square measures 0.2 mm × 0.2 mm = 0.04 mm². If five R squares are counted, then the volume used is: 5 × 0.04 mm² × 0.1 mm (depth) = 0.02 mm³. We know that 1 cc = 1 mL, therefore 1 mm³ = 1 μL:

$$\frac{1\ cm^3}{1\ mL} \times \frac{1\ mL}{1000\ \mu L} \times \frac{1000\ mm^3}{1\ cm^3} = \frac{1\ mm^3}{1\ \mu L}$$

In reality, most red cell counts are performed with a machine called a *Coulter counter* and only the white cells are counted with a haemocytometer. Let's try a problem involving white cell counts:

A blood sample is diluted $\frac{1}{100}$ and then four 'W' areas are counted on the Neubauer haemocytometer. A total of 50 cells are counted. What is the white cell count?

We can use the equation for determining the concentration of a sample that has been diluted:

Original concentration × *dilution* = *final concentration*

In these problems we are looking for the original concentration, so we can rearrange the equation:

$$Original\ concentration = \frac{final\ concentration}{dilution}$$

$$OC = \frac{\left(\dfrac{50\ cells}{4 \times 1\,mm \times 1\,mm \times 0.1\,mm}\right)}{\left(\dfrac{1}{100}\right)}$$

Number of cells counted in four 'W' squares that each has a volume of $1\,mm \times 1\,mm \times 0.1\,mm$

Dilution of original sample

$$OC = \frac{\left(\dfrac{50\ cells}{0.4\ mm^3}\right)}{\left(\dfrac{1}{100}\right)}$$

Rearrange the equation by multiplying by the reciprocal of the denominator:

$$OC = \frac{50\ cells}{0.4\ mm^3} \times \frac{100}{1}$$

$$OC = \frac{5000\ cells}{0.4\ mm^3} = \frac{12,500\ cells}{1\ mm^3}$$

Concentration of the original blood sample

In most laboratories, white cells are reported as the number of cells per litre. How do we change our value to this standard reporting method? Dimensional analysis of course!

$$\frac{12,500 \text{ cells}}{1 \text{ mm}^3} \times \frac{1 \text{ mm}^3}{1 \text{ } \mu L} \times \frac{1,000,000 \text{ } \mu L}{1 \text{ L}} = \frac{12,500,000,000 \text{ cells}}{1 \text{ L}}$$

We would use scientific notation to express such a large number, so it becomes:

1.25×10^{10} cells/L

There is another convention that says all white cell counts should be reported in such a way that the exponent is always 9. This allows the clinician to just look at the numbers to the left of the decimal point and he or she can make a quick comparison with normal values. Our white cell count expressed this way would be:

12.5×10^9 cells/L

Similarly, all red cell counts are reported with 12 as the exponent, e.g. 6.5×10^{12} cells/L.

Worlds apart

- These conventions may differ in your part of the world. Always
- convert your white and red cell counts to correspond to local
- norms in order to make comparison with normal values.

Let's do it again!

- 1. Six 'W' squares are scanned and 66 white cells are counted. The blood sample had been diluted $\frac{1}{100}$. What is the white cell count (cells/L)?

2. Four 'R' squares are scanned and 80 red cells are counted. The blood sample had been diluted $\frac{1}{100}$. What is the red cell count?

ANSWERS

1. $OC = \dfrac{\left(\dfrac{66 \text{ cells}}{6 \times 1 \text{ mm} \times 1 \text{ mm} \times 0.1 \text{ mm}}\right)}{\left(\dfrac{1}{100}\right)}$

$= \dfrac{66 \text{ cells}}{0.6 \text{ mm}^3} \times \dfrac{100}{1} = \dfrac{6600 \text{ cells}}{0.6 \text{ mm}^3}$

$= 1.1 \times 10^4 \text{ cells/mm}^3$

$= 1.1 \times 10^{10} \text{ cells/L} = 11 \times 10^9 \text{ cells/L}$

2. $OC = \dfrac{\left(\dfrac{80 \text{ cells}}{4 \times 0.2 \text{ mm} \times 0.2 \text{ mm} \times 0.1 \text{ mm}}\right)}{\left(\dfrac{1}{100}\right)} = \dfrac{80 \text{ cells}}{0.016 \text{ mm}^3} \times \dfrac{100}{1}$

$= \dfrac{8000 \text{ cells}}{0.016 \text{ mm}^3}$

$= 5 \times 10^5 \text{ cells/mm}^3 = 5 \times 10^{11} \text{ cells/L} = 0.5 \times 10^{12} \text{ cells/L}$

When using the equation: $OC \times dilution = FC$ and you are trying to find the OC, rearrange the equation into: $OC = FC \times dilution\ factor$, where *dilution factor* is the reciprocal of the dilution. For example, when the dilution is $\frac{1}{100}$, the dilution factor is 100. When the dilution is 10^{-3}, the dilution factor is 1000.

Clinical problems using dilutions

Questions

1. A 7% solution is diluted $\frac{1}{100}$. What is the final concentration?
2. How much serum would be present in 25 mL of a $\frac{1}{5}$ dilution?

3. A stock solution contains 200 g/L. What dilution is necessary to prepare a working standard containing 5 mg/100 mL?

4. You are given a series of 10 tubes, each of which contains 5 mL of diluent. To the first tube is added 1 mL of serum, and a serial dilution using 1 mL is carried out on the remaining tubes. What is the serum concentration in tubes 4 and 8?

5. You want to make 30 mL of a $\frac{1}{500}$ dilution of urine in water. How much diluent will it take?

6. After inoculating 0.5 mL of a 10^{-4} dilution on to a blood agar plate, 45 colonies are found on the plate. What is the concentration of the original solution (cfu/mL)?

7. In order to determine the quantity of bacteria in a water sample, 2 L of water was put through a filter that the organisms cannot pass through. When the filter was cultured, 15 colonies were counted. What is the concentration of organisms in the water?

8. A blood sample was first diluted $\frac{1}{100}$, then 91 white cells were counted in four 'W' areas. What is the white cell count?

9. A blood sample was first diluted $\frac{1}{20}$, then 140 cells were counted in five 'W' squares. What is the white cell count?

10. You need to dilute a drug from its original concentration of 100 mg/mL to a concentration of 0.1 mg/mL. The smallest volume you can measure accurately is 0.5 mL and the largest volume you can make at one time is 10 mL. With these restrictions, how would you make your diluted drug?

Answers

1. $OC \times dilution = FC$

$$7\% \times \frac{1}{100} = \frac{7}{100} = 0.07\%$$

2. $\dfrac{1}{5} = \dfrac{x}{25\,mL}, \quad x = 5\,mL$

Dilution is a ratio of 1 part serum to 5 parts total solution

3. $OC = 200$ g/L, $FC = 5$ mg/100 mL

$$OC \times dilution = FC, \quad Dilution = \frac{FC}{OC}$$

Since our OC and FC are in different units, we need to convert one of them into units that are the same as the other:

$$\frac{200 \, \cancel{g}}{1 \, \cancel{L}} \times \frac{1 \, \cancel{L}}{1000 \text{ mL}} \times \frac{1000 \text{ mg}}{1 \, \cancel{g}} = \frac{200 \text{ mg}}{1 \text{ mL}},$$

$$\frac{200 \text{ mg}}{1 \text{ mL}} = \frac{x \text{ mg}}{100 \text{ mL}}, \quad x = \frac{20,000 \text{ mg}}{100 \text{ mL}}$$

$$Dilution = \frac{\left(\dfrac{5 \text{ mg}}{100 \text{ mL}}\right)}{\left(\dfrac{20,000 \text{ mg}}{100 \text{ mL}}\right)} = \frac{1}{4000}$$

4. The serum began as a 100% solution and in this six-fold serial dilution it became 0.077% by the fourth tube and 0.00006% by the eighth tube (Fig. 8.5).

5. If the total volume is 30 mL, it must have the same ratio as the $\frac{1}{500}$ dilution:

$$\frac{1}{500} = \frac{x}{30 \text{ mL}}, \quad x = 0.06 \text{ mL}$$

If only 0.06 mL of the 30 mL is urine, then (30 – 0.06) 29.94 mL is diluent.

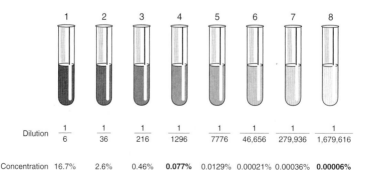

	1	2	3	4	5	6	7	8
Dilution	$\frac{1}{6}$	$\frac{1}{36}$	$\frac{1}{216}$	$\frac{1}{1296}$	$\frac{1}{7776}$	$\frac{1}{46,656}$	$\frac{1}{279,936}$	$\frac{1}{1,679,616}$
Concentration	16.7%	2.6%	0.46%	**0.077%**	0.0129%	0.00021%	0.00036%	**0.00006%**

Fig. 8.5   Dilutions for question 4

6. $OC \times dilution = FC, \quad OC = \dfrac{FC}{dilution}$

$$OC = \frac{\left(\frac{45 \text{ cfu}}{0.5 \text{ mL}}\right)}{\left(\frac{1}{10,000}\right)}, \quad OC = \frac{90 \text{ cfu}}{1 \text{ mL}} \times 10,000 = \frac{900,000 \text{ cfu}}{1 \text{ mL}},$$

$$OC = 9 \times 10^5 \text{ cfu/mL}$$

7. $\dfrac{15 \text{ cfu}}{2 \text{ L}} = \dfrac{x}{1 \text{ L}}, \quad x = 7.5 \text{ cfu/L}.$

Sometimes, it's not too complicated!

8. $OC = FC \times dilution\ factor$ (reciprocal of the dilution)

$$OC = \frac{91 \text{ cells}}{4 \times 1 \text{ mm} \times 1 \text{ mm} \times 0.1 \text{ mm}} \times 100 = \frac{9100 \text{ cells}}{0.4 \text{ mm}^3}$$

$$\frac{9100 \text{ cells}}{0.4 \text{ mm}^3} \times \frac{1 \text{ mm}^3}{1 \text{ μL}} \times \frac{1,000,000 \text{ μL}}{1 \text{ L}} = \frac{9,100,000,000 \text{ cells}}{0.4 \text{ L}}$$

$$= \frac{22,750,000,000}{1 \text{ L}}$$

$OC = 22.75 \times 10^9 \text{ cells/L}$

9. $OC = FC \times dilution\ factor$ (reciprocal of the dilution)

$$OC = \frac{140 \text{ cells}}{5 \times 1 \text{ mm} \times 1 \text{ mm} \times 0.1 \text{ mm}} \times 20 = \frac{2800 \text{ cells}}{0.5 \text{ mm}^3}$$

$$OC = \frac{2800 \text{ cells}}{0.5 \text{ mm}^3} \times \frac{1 \text{ mm}^3}{1 \text{ μL}} \times \frac{1,000,000 \text{ μL}}{1 \text{ L}}$$

$$= \frac{2,800,000,000 \text{ cells}}{0.5 \text{ L}} = \frac{5,600,000,000 \text{ cells}}{1 \text{ L}}$$

$OC = 5.6 \times 10^9 \text{ cells/L}$

10. This is a tricky problem, so let's take it one step at a time.

The dilution we require is: $\dfrac{FC}{OC} = \dfrac{0.1 \text{ mg/mL}}{100 \text{ mg/mL}} = \dfrac{1}{1000}$.

The greatest dilution we can make is limited by the smallest and largest volumes we can use. The smallest volume is 0.5 mL and the largest is 10 mL.

Therefore, the greatest dilution we can make in one step is:

$$\dfrac{0.5 \text{ mL}}{10 \text{ mL}} = \dfrac{1}{20}$$

Using a $\frac{1}{20}$ dilution as the largest dilution, how do we get to a dilution of $\frac{1}{1000}$?

We could do it several ways:

We could do three dilutions of $\frac{1}{10}$ $\left(\frac{1}{10} \times \frac{1}{10} \times \frac{1}{10} = \frac{1}{1000}\right)$, or $\frac{1}{20} \times \frac{1}{10} \times \frac{1}{5}$, or any combination to give us a $\frac{1}{1000}$ dilution within our limitations.

Multiple choice questions

1. A solution was diluted $\frac{1}{15}$ and the final concentration was 20%. What was the original concentration?
   a. 30%   b. 150%   c. 300%   d. 3000%

2. A 65% solution is diluted $\frac{7}{10}$. What is the final concentration?
   a. 37%   b. 45.5%   c. 60%   d. 55%

3. What was the original strength of the solution if it is diluted $\frac{1}{7}$ and the final concentration is 12%?
   a. 42%   b. 65%   c. 75%   d. 84%

4. A 7% solution is diluted $\frac{1}{10}$. What is the final concentration?
   a. 0.07%   b. 0.7%   c. 7%   d. 10%

5. An 80% solution was diluted to produce a 30% solution. How much was it diluted?
   a. $\frac{1}{4}$ b. $\frac{1}{3}$ c. $\frac{3}{8}$ d. $\frac{5}{8}$

Answers

1. c. 300%
2. b. 45.5%
3. d. 84%
4. b. 0.7%
5. c. $\frac{3}{8}$

Chapter 9

Anaesthesia, radiology and nutrition applications

Learning Objectives

- Calculating anaesthesia gas flow rates
- Basic radiology calculations
- Calculating nutritional requirements

Anaesthesia gas flow rates

We have performed some calculations for injectable anaesthetic agents such as propofol. Generally, these agents are used to take the patient from an awake or sedated state to a state of general anaesthesia (unconscious to most stimuli) and then a gaseous agent is administered to keep them anaesthetized. The gas is administered through an endotracheal tube, which is placed into the airway, and is delivered into the lungs where it crosses into the bloodstream and finds its way to the brain. The gas is delivered by a vaporizer that has a carrier gas (usually oxygen) that passes over the liquid anaesthetic agent and dissolves the anaesthetic into the gas.

The amount of anaesthetic gas delivered to the patient is a function of the vaporizer setting and the flow rate of carrier gas. Setting the vaporizer is simply a matter of setting the vaporizer dial to the correct percent of anaesthetic agent, but calculating the flow rate is a little more complex. Flow rates are based on the patient's size and also on the type of anaesthesia protocol. Some protocols, such as mask induction in which gas is delivered through a mask into the patient's nostrils, require a high flow rate; while others, such as maintenance on a closed circuit, require a low flow of carrier gas. We will leave it to the appropriate anaesthesia textbook to explain the different anaesthetic protocols but will use some examples to make you comfortable with the calculations.

The flow rate recommended for use just after an injectable agent has been used is equal to the *respiratory minute volume* (*RMV*). The RMV is equal to the tidal volume (the volume of a normal inhalation) multiplied by the respiratory rate, which averages about 20 breaths per minute. The tidal volume varies with the size of the animal and is calculated at about 10 mL/kg. A 30-kg Labrador retriever would, therefore, have a tidal volume of 300 mL – in other words, in each normal breath about 300 mL of air is exchanged.

Calculate the correct anaesthesia gas flow rate following injectable induction for a 20-kg dog.

Flow rate = *Respiratory minute volume*

Flow rate = *Tidal volume* × *Respiratory rate*

Flow rate = 10 mL/kg × 20/min

$$Flow\ rate = 20\ \cancel{kg} \times \frac{10\ mL}{1\ \cancel{kg}} \times \frac{20}{min} = \frac{4000\ mL}{min}$$

The flow rate recommended for mask induction (where no injectable agent is used) is 30 times the tidal volume.

Calculate the flow rate required for mask induction of a 4-kg cat.

Flow rate = 30 × *Tidal volume*

Flow rate = 30 × 10 mL/kg

$$Flow\ rate = 4\ \cancel{kg} \times \frac{10\ mL}{\cancel{kg}} \times 30 = 1200\ mL\ (per\ minute)$$

The lowest flow rate that can be given to an animal is its metabolic oxygen needs – enough to provide for resting metabolism. In small animals under anaesthesia, this value is 15 mL/kg/min. What is the lowest flow rate that you could give to the 20-kg dog above?

Flow rate = 15 mL/kg/min

$$Flow\ rate = \frac{15\ mL}{1\ \cancel{kg}} \times 20\ \cancel{kg} = 300\ mL\ \text{(per minute)}$$

Flow rate calculations can vary according to the anaesthetic protocol and there is considerable leeway for the clinician's own judgement, but dimensional analysis is a good tool for coming up with the correct amount.

Radiology calculations

Although modern technology has created x-ray machines that are fully automated, there are some basic calculations that veterinary nurses and technicians should understand.

X-rays are created when electrons are energized, escape their orbits from the atoms of the material to which they belong and collide with a second material, producing photons. The amount of x-rays produced depends on the number of electrons freed from their orbits, which is directly linked to the amount of energy applied to the first material, and this is measured in milliamperes (mA). As more energy (milliamperage) is applied, more electrons are available and the intensity of the x-ray beam is increased.

The image on the x-ray film is produced when these electrons pass through the object being x-rayed and interact with the film or digital receptor. Once developed, the film or digital image will be black where the electrons interact with the film or receptor and white where the electrons were blocked by the object being x-rayed. Thus a bone appears white because the dense material in the bone prevented the electrons from striking the film or digital receptor.

The total quantity of x-rays produced during a given exposure will depend on the milliamperage (mA) and the duration of the exposure (fractions of a second). We can therefore vary the quantity of x-rays produced in a given exposure by adjusting the milliamperage or the duration of the exposure. This quantity is expressed as milliamperage-seconds (mAs).

Consider the examples below, which all produce the same total amount of x-rays:

$$20 \text{ mA} \times \frac{1}{2} \text{ s} = 10 \text{ mAs}$$

$$100 \text{ mA} \times \frac{1}{10} \text{ s} = 10 \text{ mAs}$$

$$200 \text{ mA} \times \frac{1}{20} \text{ s} = 10 \text{ mAs}$$

$$300 \text{ mA} \times \frac{1}{30} \text{ s} = 10 \text{ mAs}$$

Using a higher mA is advantageous, as it allows a reduction in exposure time. This lessens the chance that the animal will move and create a blurry image and also cuts down the exposure to the restraining personnel. Today's digital radiography equipment automates most functions but it is useful to understand the basic fundamentals.

Nutritional calculations

Veterinary technicians are often required to calculate the nutritional needs of patients, both for normal activity and for therapeutic situations such as recovering from illness. The basis for nutritional calculations is determining the *energy requirements* of the patient. This assumes that a *balanced* diet is fed in which, once the energy requirements are determined, all other nutrients are present in the correct amounts.

The unit used for determining energy requirements is the *calorie*, which is defined as the amount of energy needed to raise

1 mL of water from 14.5°C to 15.5°C. There are 1000 calories in 1 kilocalorie (kcal). When people talk about the number of calories in the food they consume, they are actually referring to kcal or 1000 calories. The energy density of foods is determined by dividing the kcal present in the food by the weight of the food (kcal/g).

Animals require varying levels of nutrition depending on their physical state. A healthy cat sitting in a kennel requires much less energy than one chasing mice outside. We need a system to determine these different needs.

 ## Worlds apart

There are different systems for calculating the basic requirements for energy needs. Some use the term *metabolizable energy requirements* (MER) for the needs of a healthy animal at rest, whereas others use the term *resting energy requirements* (RER). Consult a nutritional reference for your needs and apply the principles presented below.

Resting energy requirement

This term is used for the energy needs of a healthy animal at rest in a thermoneutral environment – in other words in a warm kennel. The RER is calculated by using the *ideal body weight* (BW) of the patient in the formula:

$$30 \times BW \text{ (in kg)} + 70$$

For a 10-kg dog, the RER would be: $30 \times 10 \text{ kg} + 70 = 370$ kcal.

The RER is then adjusted based on the activity level or therapeutic needs of the patient. Table 9.1 is one suggested guide.

Table 9.1 Multipliers for the resting energy requirement (RER)

Active or therapeutic state	Multiply RER by
Maintenance	1.2
Growth	1.5–2
Moderate activity	1.25
Very active	2
Weight loss	0.8
Pregnant (last trimester)	1.3
Lactating (peak)	3–4
Post surgery	1.5
Major infection	2

Let's do it again!

1. What is the RMV of a 10-kg dog breathing at 15 breaths per minute?
2. If you had to use mask induction to anaesthetize the 10-kg dog in question 1, what flow rate would you use?
3. What is the lowest flow rate to meet the oxygen requirements of the 10-kg dog?
4. You are asked to set the x-ray machine to produce 40 mAs. Using a setting of 200 mA, what will be your exposure time?
5. To create the same exposure as in question 4 with a machine that can only produce 40 mA, what will be your exposure time?
6. What are the energy requirements for a 22-kg Labrador retriever that runs 10 km with its owner every day?
7. How much energy does an obese 7-kg cat that should weigh 4 kg require?
8. Calculate the energy needs of a 60-lb German Shepherd following surgery to stabilize a torn ligament in its knee joint.
9. A 12-lb cat that is moderately active is fed a food with a caloric density of 380 kcal per cup. How many cups per day should it be fed?

ANSWERS

1. $RMV = Tidal\ volume \times Respiratory\ rate$

$$= \left(\frac{10\ mL}{kg} \times 10\ kg\right) \times \left(\frac{15\ breaths}{min}\right) = 1500\ mL/min$$

2. Flow rate for mask induction $= 30 \times$ tidal volume

$$30 \times 10\,\frac{mL}{kg} \times 10\ kg = 3000\ mL$$

3. Metabolic oxygen needs $= 15\,\dfrac{mL}{kg\text{-}min}$

$$= 15\,\frac{mL}{1\ kg\text{-}min} \times 10\ kg = 150\ mL/min$$

4. $mAs = mA \times seconds$

   $Seconds = \dfrac{mAs}{mA}$

   $Seconds = \dfrac{40\ mAs}{200\ mA} = \dfrac{1}{5}$ seconds

5. $Seconds = \dfrac{mAs}{mA} = \dfrac{40\ mAs}{40\ mA} = 1$ second

6. $Energy = 2 \times RER$
   $Energy = 2 \times [(30 \times 22\ kg) + 70]$
   $Energy = 1460\ kcal$

7. $Energy = 0.8 \times RER$
   $Energy = 0.8 \times [(30 \times 4) + 70]$
   $Energy = 152\ kcal$

8. $Energy = 1.5 \times RER$

$$Energy = 1.5 \times \left\{\left[30 \times \left(60\ lb \times \frac{1\ kg}{2.2\ lb}\right)\right] + 70\right\}$$

$Energy = 1332\ kcal$

Note that we had to convert the patient's weight from pounds to kilograms in order to use our energy formula.

9. Weight in kg: $12 \text{ lb} \times \dfrac{1 \text{ kg}}{2.2 \text{ lb}} = 5.45 \text{ kg}$

30 (5.45 kg) + 70 = 234 kcal RER × 1.25 for moderately active = 294 kcal required

$294 \text{ kcal} \times \dfrac{1 \text{ cup}}{380 \text{ kcal}} = 0.8 \text{ cups}$

Multiple choice questions

1. Calculate the RER for a 24.6-kg dog.
   a. 560 kcal   b. 607 kcal   c. 808 kcal   d. 924 kcal

2. A 7-kg puppy still requires the energy requirement for growth. How many kcal does it need per day?
   a. 290 kcal   b. 360 kcal   c. 420 kcal   d. 560 kcal

3. Calculate the energy needs of a 10-kg dog that requires one and a half times its RER.
   a. 155 kcal   b. 310 kcal   c. 555 kcal   d. 930 kcal

4. A 26.5-kg dog should ideally weigh 17 kg. What is the recommended energy requirement to assist weight loss?
   a. 221 kcal   b. 316 kcal   c. 464 kcal   d. 553 kcal

5. An 18.7-kg Border Collie is in the last trimester of pregnancy. Calculate her RER.
   a. 820.3 kcal   b. 741.4 kcal   c. 635.5 kcal   d. 521.6 kcal

Answers

1. c. 808 kcal
2. d. 560 kcal
3. c. 555 kcal
4. c. 464 kcal
5. a. 820.3 kcal

Chapter 10

Statistics and quality control

Learning Objectives

- Understanding measures of central tendency
- Understanding distribution, ranges and variance
- Calculating standard deviation
- Using statistics in quality control

Basic knowledge of statistics is very useful in the veterinary clinic and essential in the veterinary research laboratory. It helps us to quickly determine if something is strange or unusual compared to what we might expect such as the weight of a basset hound and when it comes to quality control, it is needed to ensure equipment is functioning properly.

Measures of central tendency

Whenever we are presented with a lot of information, it's nice to be able to summarize it somehow – to 'get to the heart of the matter' or see a 'snapshot' in order to be able to understand the essence of the information quickly. Working with numerical information is no different: we like to get an *average* value to help us understand it. An average reduces many individual pieces of information to a single 'typical' value. While we all have a general idea what *average* means, there are actually three different types of average used scientifically.

Mean

The mean is the arithmetical average of a set of values – to get the mean, add up all the values and divide by the number of values. It can be expressed as:

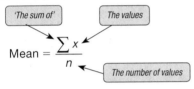

$$\text{Mean} = \frac{\sum x}{n}$$

'The sum of' The values The number of values

If we had test scores of 60, 65, 70, 75, 80, then the mean would be:

$$\text{Mean} = \frac{60 + 65 + 70 + 75 + 80}{5} = 70$$

The mean is the most reliable of the averages when the values we are evaluating form a *normal distribution*.

Median

The median is the number that divides the data in half, with the same number of values appearing on either side of the median. For example, if the scores on an exam are 60, 65, 70, 75, 80, 85, 90, then the median score is 75, as there are three scores on either side. On another exam the scores are 60, 60, 65, 68, 72, 78, 78, 80, 90. The median score here is 72, as there are four scores on either side.

What if there is an even number of values so that there is no 'middle' value? In that case the two middle values are added

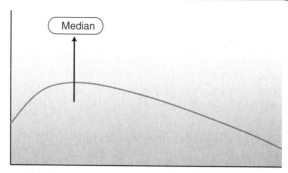

Fig. 10.1 This is a skewed set of data: more values occur towards one end of the distribution than the other

together and divided by two. Here's another set of test scores: 65, 68, 70, 74, 80, 85. In this case, 70 and 74 are the two middle scores so the median is $\frac{(70+74)}{2} = 72$.

The median is useful to describe a set of values that do not form a normal distribution but are *skewed*, i.e. more values occur towards one end of the distribution than the other (Fig. 10.1).

An example of using the median to describe a set of values could be found in a class of veterinary technicians, in which the age of the students may vary from, for instance, 17 to 57. Let's say this is your class and most of your classmates are between 18 and 24, but there are two people who are in their 30s and one in her 50s. The graph of the distribution of the ages of the class would resemble the one in Fig. 10.1. The mean value of the class would be pulled higher by the three more mature class members, but it would not really be a good picture of the age of most of the class members. In this case, the median would describe the class age more accurately.

Mode

The mode is the value that occurs most often. This is the easiest value to find but it can be misleading. The mode is not used often in the clinical setting.

Normal distribution

The so-called *bell curve* of normal distribution is familiar to students who are ranked according to how well each member of the class performs. Values are plotted from lowest to highest and the most common values will be found in the middle of the distribution (Fig. 10.2).

The mean of the values will be in centre of the distribution. In other words, the area under the curve on one side of the mean will equal the area under the curve on the other side of the mean. Many sets of measured values will form a normal curve as, in many different situations where things are measured, it is usual to have a few very low values and a few very high values, with most values falling somewhere near the middle. One example would be white blood cell counts in a healthy population of dogs.

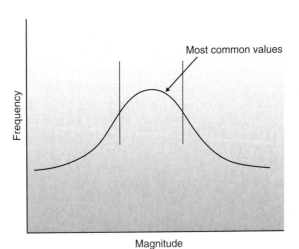

Fig. 10.2 A typical bell curve. The magnitude of each value is on the horizontal axis and the frequency on the vertical axis. The most common values are found near the middle of the curve

Variance

When we examine a normal distribution of values we see that, while most values fall near the middle, some values are very low and some very high. The more of these low and high values we have, the greater is the variance. A good snapshot of the variance of a set of values can be obtained by looking at the *range* – the difference between the lowest value and the highest. If a set of test scores is 50, 53, 58, 65, 73, 83, 90, then the range is 90 − 50 = 40. Another set might be 65, 68, 71, 75, 81, 82, 88 and the range would be 88 − 65 = 23. The range of the second set is smaller than the first – in other words, there is *less variance*. There is an expected variance for any set of values that has a normal distribution, so we need a way to evaluate how one value compares with the expected values – this is the *standard deviation*.

Standard deviation

We have learned that the mean is the arithmetical average of the values. The standard deviation is the *arithmetical average of the variations from the mean*. It tells us how likely it is for a value to fall close to the mean of the values. Consider a series of blood glucose tests done on healthy dogs. We could plot all the test results and, if we had enough values, they would form a normal distribution (Fig. 10.3). Now suppose I take another blood glucose test from a dog that comes into the clinic. I would like to know if this dog's test result is 'normal' – is it an expected result in a healthy dog?

I can take this value and see where it falls on my normal distribution created earlier. If it is near the middle then I know it's normal. If it's near one of the ends of the curve, it *may* be abnormal.

 The standard deviation is a guide to tell us how far from the middle a value should be before it is considered abnormal.

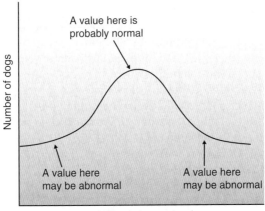

Fig. 10.3 Blood glucose measurements from dogs. How exactly do we know when values are normal or abnormal? The answer is to use the standard deviation

Table 10.1	Blood glucose results from 12 dogs										
Dog	1	2	3	4	5	6	7	8	9	10	11	12
Glucose (mmol/L)	3.8	4.1	4.3	2.9	3.2	4.6	4.3	3.9	4.9	3.8	4.1	5.1

The standard deviation is calculated by first finding the mean and then finding the average of all the differences from the mean. Since some values are less than the mean, their difference from the mean will be negative; for this reason, to eliminate the negatives, we use a squaring technique, followed by finding the square root. Let's look at an example to illustrate this.

Blood glucose of 12 healthy dogs was measured and the values are listed in Table 10.1.

The mean value is:

$$\frac{\left[3.8 + 4.1 + 4.3 + 2.9 + 3.2 + 4.6 + 4.3 + 3.9 + 4.9 + 3.8 + 4.1 + 5.1\right]}{12}$$

Table 10.2   Squares of deviation from the mean blood glucose result

Value (x)	Mean ($\bar{x}$)	Variation from mean ($x - \bar{x}$)	Square of variation ($x - \bar{x}$)^2
3.8	4.1	−0.3	0.09
4.1	4.1	0	0
4.3	4.1	+0.2	0.04
2.9	4.1	−1.2	1.44
3.2	4.1	−0.9	0.81
4.6	4.1	+0.5	0.25
4.3	4.1	+0.2	0.04
3.9	4.1	−0.2	0.04
4.9	4.1	+0.8	0.64
3.8	4.1	−0.3	0.09
4.1	4.1	0	0
5.1	4.1	1	1

$$\sum (x - \bar{x})^2 = 4.44$$

Mean $(\bar{x}) = 4.08$. Let's round to the nearest one-tenth and call the mean 4.1.

The next step (Table 10.2) is to total the squares of the deviation from the mean:

> Σ is the symbol for 'the sum of'

$$\sum (x - \bar{x})^2 = 4.44$$

We then divide this total by the number of values minus one $(n − 1)$. The reason for using one less than the total number of values is a statistical parameter known as *degrees of freedom*. This is related to the fact that, since we used the original values to come up with the mean, and then *used* the mean to come up with another value, we have used up 'one degree of freedom' and must therefore subtract 1 from the number of values. (You don't need to worry about the statistical theory behind this.)

This number is called the variance, s^2, and can be expressed as:

$$\frac{\sum(x - \bar{x})}{(n-1)}$$

In this case:

$$s^2 = \frac{4.44}{11} = 0.40$$

Since we used the *square* of the differences between the mean and each value to determine the variance, if we now take the *square root* of the variance, we arrive at the standard deviation, abbreviated s:

$$s = \sqrt{s^2}, \quad s = \sqrt{0.40} = 0.63$$

If we look back at the stages of getting to this value, we see that the complete formula for the standard deviation can be shown as:

$$s = \sqrt{\frac{\sum(x - \bar{x})^2}{(n-1)}}$$

Given this set of healthy dogs, we have determined the mean blood glucose value is 4.1 mmol/L, with a standard deviation of 0.63 mmol/L. If we were to measure another dog's blood glucose and find it to be 6.3 mmol/L, we would now know that the value is too high to be considered normal, as it falls beyond 2 standard deviations of the mean (more of this later).

 Let's do it again!

- Find the mean and standard deviation for the following.

- 1. A set of exam scores: 48, 51, 53, 59, 61, 66, 70, 71, 76, 78, 81, 82, 88, 91, 99.

2. Ages of students in a class: 17, 18, 19, 19, 20, 20, 20, 21, 21, 22, 22, 23, 25, 25, 26, 34, 48.
3. White cell counts in healthy cats (all are $\times 10^9$ cells/L): 5.2, 3.9, 4.5, 6.3, 6.8, 7.9, 4.9, 10.2, 9.3, 11.4, 12.5, 8.1, 6.7.

ANSWERS

1. The data are given in Table 10.3.

$$s = \sqrt{\frac{\sum(x - \bar{x})^2}{(n-1)}}, \quad s = \sqrt{\frac{3285.60}{14}}, \quad s = 15.32$$

The mean test score is 71.6, with a standard deviation of 15.32.

Table 10.3 Exam scores (question 1)

Value (x)	Mean ($\bar{x}$)	Variation from mean ($x - \bar{x}$)	Square of variation ($x - \bar{x}$)^2
48	71.6	−23.6	556.96
51	71.6	−20.6	424.36
53	71.6	−18.6	345.96
59	71.6	−12.6	158.76
61	71.6	−10.6	112.36
66	71.6	−5.6	31.36
70	71.6	−1.6	2.56
71	71.6	−0.6	0.36
76	71.6	4.4	19.36
78	71.6	6.4	40.96
81	71.6	9.4	88.36
82	71.6	10.4	108.16
88	71.6	16.4	268.96
91	71.6	19.4	376.36
99	71.6	27.4	750.76
			$\sum(x - \bar{x}) = 3285.60$

2. The data are given in Table 10.4.

$$s = \sqrt{\frac{\sum(x - \bar{x})^2}{(n - 1)}}, \quad s = \sqrt{\frac{888.24}{16}}, \quad s = 7.45$$

The mean age of the class is 23.5 years, with a standard deviation of 7.45 years. Note that this is not a normal distribution of values – it is skewed by the two older students. This means the 'average' age is not really a good snapshot of the class as a whole and that the standard deviation is not a helpful value in this case.

Table 10.4 Student ages (question 2)			
Value (x)	Mean ($\bar{x}$)	Variation from mean ($x - $)	Square of variation ($x - $)^2
17	23.5	−6.5	42.63
18	23.5	−5.5	30.57
19	23.5	−4.5	20.52
19	23.5	−4.5	20.52
20	23.5	−3.5	12.46
20	23.5	−3.5	12.46
20	23.5	−3.5	12.46
21	23.5	−2.5	6.40
21	23.5	−2.5	6.40
22	23.5	−1.5	2.34
22	23.5	−1.5	2.34
23	23.5	−0.5	0.28
25	23.5	1.5	2.16
25	23.5	1.5	2.16
26	23.5	2.5	6.10
34	23.5	10.5	109.63
48	23.5	24.5	598.81
			$\sum(x - \bar{x}) = 888.24$

3. The data are given in Table 10.5.

$$s = \sqrt{\frac{\sum(x - \bar{x})^2}{(n-1)}}, \quad s = \sqrt{\frac{87.84}{12}}, \quad s = 2.71$$

The mean white cell count is 7.5×10^9, with a standard deviation of 2.71×10^9 cells/L.

Table 10.5 White cell counts in cats (3×10^9 cells/L) (question 3)

Value (x)	Mean ($\bar{x}$)	Variation from mean ($x - \bar{x}$)	Square of variation ($x - \bar{x}$)^2
5.2	7.5	−2.3	5.36
3.9	7.5	−3.6	13.07
4.5	7.5	−3.0	9.09
6.3	7.5	−1.2	1.48
6.8	7.5	−0.7	0.51
7.9	7.5	0.4	0.15
4.9	7.5	−2.6	6.84
10.2	7.5	2.7	7.21
9.3	7.5	1.8	3.18
11.4	7.5	3.9	15.09
12.5	7.5	5.0	24.85
8.1	7.5	0.6	0.34
6.7	7.5	−0.8	0.66
			$\sum(x - \bar{x}) = 87.84$

Using the normal curve

As we have seen, when a set of data forms a normal distribution, there are equal numbers on either side of the mean and the mean is the most common value – the highest point on the curve.

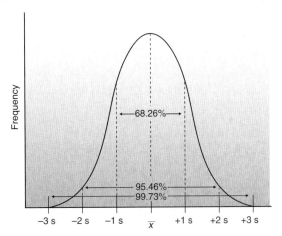

Fig. 10.4 The curve of normal distribution

All values fall between the two points on the curve but the most common values will be found near the middle, close to the mean. The standard deviation calculation tells us how likely it is that a value will fall in between two points on the curve. Fig. 10.4 shows that, on any normal curve, 68.26% of the values will fall between −1 and +1 standard deviations from the mean, 95.46% will fall between −2 and +2 standard deviations, and virtually all values will fall between −3 and +3 standard deviations from the mean.

When considering a value derived from a clinical test, we can compare it to a normal curve and see if it is within an acceptable range. For most clinical tests, a value that falls within ±2 standard deviations is considered normal. The normal curve was first created using data from a large set of healthy individuals and then determining the mean and standard deviation. Let's look at an example.

A laboratory was setting up its reference ranges for sodium values in healthy dogs. A total of 100 dogs were sampled and the mean value was 145 mmol/L with a standard deviation of 2.5 mmol/L. What was the reference range for healthy dogs?

If the reference range is ±2 standard deviations, then the reference range is:

$$145 - (2 \times 2.5) = 140 \, \text{mmol/L to} \, 145 + (2 \times 2.5)$$
$$= 150 \, \text{mmol/L}$$

If a dog's blood was found to have a value of 135 mmol/L of sodium, it would be considered abnormally low.

Barking up the wrong tree

If a value falls below 2 standard deviations on a clinical test it is considered abnormal but it may, in fact, be normal for that individual. Remember that ±2 standard deviations encompasses 95.46% of the 'normal' values. It may be that this 'abnormal' value is one of the 4.54% *outside* the 2 standard deviations. This is why it is important to look at the patient as well as the clinical test results!

Statistics and quality control

When performing a clinical test such as measuring blood glucose, how can you be assured that the test procedure and equipment are reliable? After all, if *they* are unreliable, the test result is also unreliable. Quality control charts are used to ensure reliability of this type and can tell the operator when a particular test is 'out of control'. These charts are called Levey–Jennings charts. These are created by conducting a series of control tests and then plotting a normal curve and outlining the standard deviations (Fig. 10.5). Note that the normal curve has been 'turned sideways'.

The Levey–Jennings chart is then used to assess a control test each day (or at whatever time interval the laboratory deems adequate). If the control test falls within 2 standard deviations, then the test is considered *in control* (the control solution, equipment and procedure are all behaving the way they should). If the control

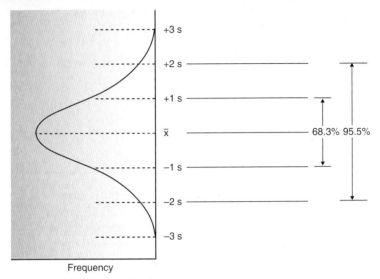

Frequency

Fig. 10.5   The Levey–Jennings chart

test falls outside that range, the control test is repeated; if it then falls within 2 standard deviations, the test is considered in control. If the second test also falls outside the 2 standard deviations, the test is considered *out of control* and the problem must be identified. It may be a problem with the control solution, the testing equipment or the procedure.

Let's see how a Levey–Jennings chart is created. Let's imagine that a chemistry analyser used in a veterinary clinic comes with control solutions that have a value assigned to them from the manufacturer. In our example, we will use blood glucose that has a control value of 4.5 mmol/L. For the month of March, the control solution was taken out each day and tested on the chemistry analyser. The results were tabulated and a mean and standard deviation calculated, as shown in Table 10.6.

The control solution has an assigned value of 4.5 mmol/L. Each day, it is measured and a value recorded. Since the procedure and equipment are going to have *some* random variability, we must

Table 10.6   Blood glucose test control figures (March)

Day	(x)	(x −)	(x −)²
1	4.6	0	0
2	4.4	−0.2	0.04
3	4.8	0.2	0.02
4	4.5	−0.1	0.01
5	3.9	−0.7	0.49
6	5.1	0.5	0.25
7	5.0	0.4	0.16
8	4.9	0.3	0.09
9	3.9	−0.7	0.49
10	4.4	−0.2	0.04
11	4.7	0.1	0.01
12	4.5	−0.1	0.01
13	5.0	0.4	0.16
14	5.1	0.5	0.25
15	4.4	−0.2	0.04
16	4.3	−0.3	0.09
17	4.7	0.1	0.01
18	4.8	0.2	0.04
19	4.3	−0.3	0.09
20	4.7	0.1	0.01
21	4.1	−0.5	0.25
22	5.0	0.5	0.25
23	4.8	0.2	0.04
24	4.3	−0.3	0.09
25	4.7	0.1	0.01
26	4.3	−0.3	0.09
27	4.9	0.3	0.09
28	4.2	−0.4	0.16
29	4.2	−0.4	0.04

Continued

Table 10.6 Blood glucose test control figures (March)

Day	(x)	(x –)	(x –)²
30	4.7	0.1	0.01
31	4.8	0.2	0.04
	$\bar{x} = 4.6$		$\sum (x - \bar{x})^2 = 3.37$

determine the mean of the values and the standard deviation for our laboratory.

The mean is calculated to be 4.6 mmol/L with a standard deviation of:

$$s = \sqrt{\frac{(x - \bar{x})^2}{N - 1}}$$

$$s = \sqrt{\frac{3.37}{30}} = 0.34$$

With this information, we can create our Levey–Jennings chart, which we can start using in April.

In the month of April, we will test our control solution on our equipment. If the reading is between 3.92 and 5.28 (4.6 ± 2 standard deviations), then we say the test is in control and we can carry on measuring blood samples that day. If the control solution falls below or above this range, we must repeat it; if it is still outside the range, we must determine why the test is out of control.

There are two other situations in which a test may be considered out of control: when the control test results have a number of values in a row that fall on one side of the mean, or when a series of consecutive values forms a line in one direction. We call the first case a *shift* – the mean has shifted up or down; the second case is called a *trend* – there is something causing the values of the control solution to increase or decrease each day. The acceptable number of consecutive values on one side of the mean or the number going in one direction varies in each laboratory but six is a commonly used number, i.e. action must be taken when six such readings are obtained. Figs 10.6 and 10.7 illustrate a shift and a trend.

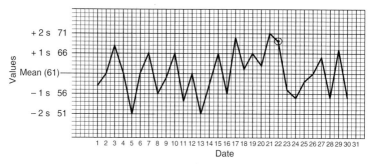

Fig. 10.6 A shift: from the 17th until the 22nd there are six consecutive readings above the mean

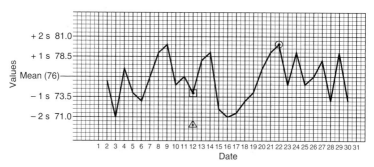

Fig. 10.7 A trend: showing a consecutive increase in readings for 7 days between the 16th and 22nd

 You may find some variation on the detail of quality control procedures as used from laboratory to laboratory, but remember two things about testing: your test result is only as reliable as the test itself and always look at the patient – not just the numbers!

Multiple choice questions

The table below shows a cat's glucose results taken over 11 hours.

Hour 1	9.2
Hour 2	8.4
Hour 3	3.3
Hour 4	5.4
Hour 5	7.4
Hour 6	8.4
Hour 7	4.2
Hour 8	4.8
Hour 9	4.8
Hour 10	4.8
Hour 11	5.1

1. What is the mode?
   a. 4.8   b. 5.4   c. 8.4   d. 8.8

2. What is the median?
   a. 3.8   b. 5.1   c. 7.3   d. 9.2

3. What is the mean?
   a. 5.05   b. 6   c. 7.15   d. 8.8

4. What is the range?
   a. 3.3   b. 4.8   c. 5.5   d. 5.9

5. What is the standard deviation?
   a. 1.9   b. 2.09   c. 2.12   d. 2.5

Answers

1. a. 4.8
2. b. 5.1
3. b. 6
4. d. 5.9
5. a. 1.9

Index

Note: Page numbers followed by *f* indicate figures, *t* indicate tables, and *b* indicate boxes.